Pharmaceutical Microbiology I

Zankhana P Sheth M Pharm, PhD
Assistant Professor
Sat Kaival College of Pharmacy, Sarsa, Gujarat

Amish A Dangi M Pharm, PhD
Assistant Professor
B Pharmacy College, Navalgadh
Avantika Education Trust, Dhanagadhra
Ahemadabad

M M Soniwala M Pharm, PhD
Associate Professor
B K Mody Government Pharmacy College, Rajkot

Punit Rachh M Pharm, PhD
Head, R & D
Mehta Group of Companies, Rajkot

W0193028

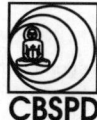

CBSPD

CBS Publishers & Distributors Pvt Ltd

New Delhi • Bengaluru • Chennai • Kochi • Kolkata • Lucknow • Mumbai
Hyderabad • Jharkhand • Nagpur • Patna • Pune • Uttarakhand

Pharmaceutical Microbiology I

ISBN: 978-81-239-2511-0

Copyright © Authors and Publisher

First Edition: 2015

Reprint: 2018, 2019, 2023

Published by Satish Kumar Jain and produced by Varun Jain for

CBS Publishers & Distributors Pvt Ltd

4819/XI Prahlad Street, 24 Ansari Road, Daryaganj, New Delhi 110 002, India
Ph: 011-23289259, 23266861, 23266867   Website: www.cbspd.com
Fax: 011-23243014   e-mail: delhi@cbspd.com; cbspubs@airtelmail.in
Corporate Office: 204 FIE, Industrial Area, Patparganj, Delhi 110 092
Ph: 011-4934 4934   Fax: 011-4934 4935   e-mail: publishing@cbspd.com;
                                            publicity@cbspd.com

Branches

- **Bengaluru:** Seema House 2975, 17th Cross, KR Road, Banasankari 2nd Stage, Bengaluru 560 070, Karnataka, India
  Ph: +91-80-26771678/79   Fax: +91-80-26771680   e-mail: bangalore@cbspd.com
- **Chennai:** 7, Subbaraya Street, Shenoy Nagar, Chennai 600 030, Tamil Nadu, India
  Ph: +91-44-26680620, 26681266   Fax: +91-44-42032115   e-mail: chennai@cbspd.com
- **Kochi:** 42/1325, 1326, Power House Road, Opp KSEB, Power House, Ernakulam 682 018, India
  Ph: +91-484-4059061-65   Fax: +91-484-4059065   e-mail: kochi@cbspd.com
- **Kolkata:** 147, Hind Ceramics Compound, 1st Floor, Nilgunj Road, Belghoria, Kolkata 700 056, West Bengal, India
  Ph: +91-9096713055/56   e-mail: kolkata@cbspd.com
- **Lucknow:** Basement, Khushnuma Complex, 7-Meerabai Marg (behind Jawahar Bhawan), Lucknow 226 001, India
  Ph: +91-522-4000032   e-mail: tiwari.lucknow@cbspd.com
- **Mumbai:** PWD Shed. Gala no. 25/26, Ramchandra Bhatt Marg, Next to JJ Hospital Gate no. 2, Opp. Union Bank of India, Noorbaug Mumbai 400 009, Maharashtra, India
  Ph: +91-22-66661880/89   e-mail: mumbai@cbspd.com

Representatives

- **Hyderabad** 0-9885175004 • **Jharkhand** 0-9811541605 • **Nagpur** 0-9421945513
- **Patna** 0-9334159340 • **Pune** 0-9623451994 • **Uttarakhand** 0-9716462459

Printed at SRK Graphics, Delhi, India

Preface

Microbiology is a very large and multifaceted field that interfaces with and stimulates research study in many peripheral fields such as bacteriology, virology, mycology, taxonomy of actinomycetes, rickettsia, identification techniques of organisms, dynamics and evaluation of disinfection, advanced sterilization technique, analytical microbiology, etc. Our motivation to write about the *Pharmaceutical Microbiology I* guided us in defining the scope of microbiology in recent age. In making this decision, we did not emphasize only the area related to bacteriology or virology. Our motivation to write this book is to cover all the areas of microbiology which help the students, teachers, academician, industrial analysts, microbiologists, researchers, etc. Many of these peripheral areas are brought into the discussion. The contents are organized with the following chapters:

- Introduction to Scope of Microbiology
- General Microbiology
- Control of Microbes
- Analytical Microbiology

In Chapter 1 we define the scope of the microbiology in detail. We begin with introduction, classification of microorganisms, historical background of microbiology, application and future of microbiology. We continue with an overview of bacteriology, virology, rickettsia, actinomycetes, etc. in Chapter 2. In Chapter 3 we have discussed different terms used to control the microorganisms and various sterilization methods and, in Chapter 4 we have highlighted analytical microbiology, sterility testing and microbiological assay methods.

We chose to proceed with the publication because we prefer to have a book in print than one perpetually in

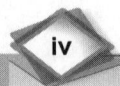

preparation. In a work such as this, there are bound to be oversights and mistakes, and we take full responsibility for them. We are receptive to readers' comments and suggestions for improvement, including updating. If the book has a second printing, we will attempt to incorporate corrections and suggestions. It has not been possible to provide complete referencing of all the significant chapters of microbiology.

We are thankful to B Pharmacy College, Navalgadh, run by Avantika Education Trust, Sat Kaival College of Pharmacy, BK Mody Govt. Pharmacy College and Atmiya Institute of Pharmacy for providing professional approach. We are immensely grateful to Param Pujya Shri Avichaldas Maharaj for his blessings and Dr Bhagirath K Patel (Principal, Sat Kaival College of Pharmacy) for his excellent guidance. We are thankful to Mr Mehulbhai H Patel, President, B Pharmacy College, Navalgadh, for providing financial support for this book. Also, we are equally thankful to Dr J R Chawda (Principal, BK Mody Govt. Pharmacy College) for his valuable suggestions. We are also thankful to Mr Gautam H Mehta (Director, Mehta Group of Companies) for his flowless inspiration. We appreciate the cooperation and interest shown by Mr YN Arjuna (Sr Vice-President—Publishing, Editorial and Publicity) and Mr Deepak Rao of CBS Publishers and Distributors (P) Ltd for publishing this book. Suggestions from students and colleagues around the world have been most helpful in the formulation of this book.

Zankhana P Sheth
Amish A Dangi
M M Soniwala
Punit Rachh

Contents

Preface   v

1. Introduction to Scope of Microbiology   1

2. General Microbiology   19

3. Control of Microbes   129

4. Analytical Microbiology   210

Bibliography   275

Index   277

Plate 1

Phase contrast light pathways

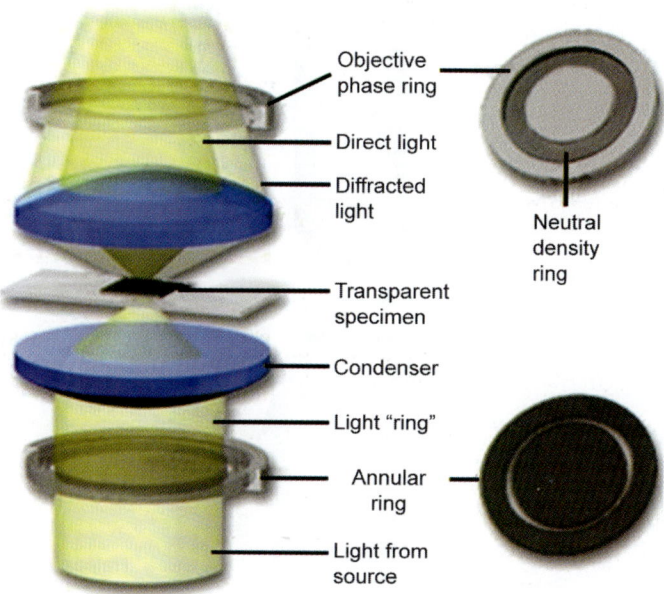

- Objective phase ring
- Direct light
- Diffracted light
- Neutral density ring
- Transparent specimen
- Condenser
- Light "ring"
- Annular ring
- Light from source

Fig. 2.5: Phase contrast microscopy

Plate 2

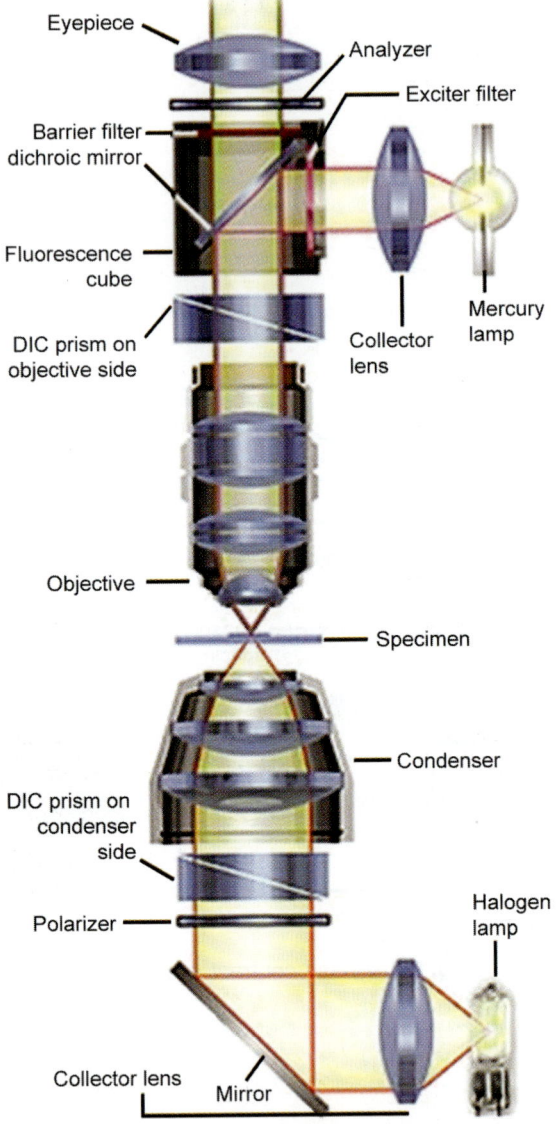

Fig. 2.6: Differential interference contrast (DIC) microscopy

Plate 3

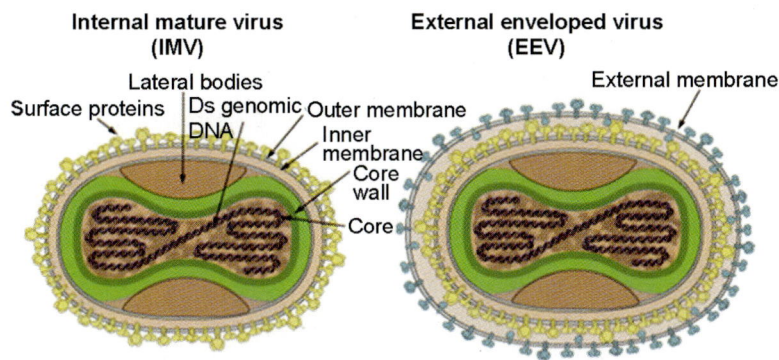

Internal mature virus (IMV)

Lateral bodies
Surface proteins
Ds genomic DNA
Outer membrane
Inner membrane
Core wall
Core

External enveloped virus (EEV)

External membrane

Fig. 2.44: Structure of enveloped viruses

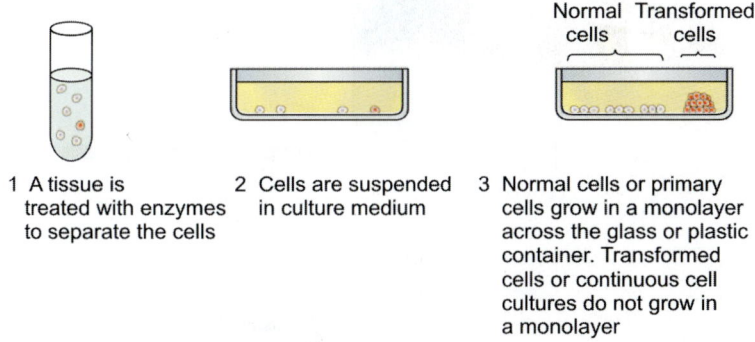

Normal cells   Transformed cells

1 A tissue is treated with enzymes to separate the cells

2 Cells are suspended in culture medium

3 Normal cells or primary cells grow in a monolayer across the glass or plastic container. Transformed cells or continuous cell cultures do not grow in a monolayer

Fig. 2.50: Continuous cell lines

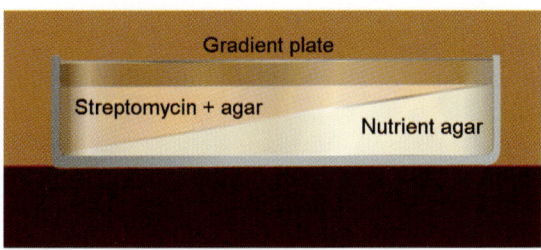

Gradient plate

Streptomycin + agar

Nutrient agar

Fig. 3.17: Assessment of bacteriostatic activity by gradient plate method

Plate 4

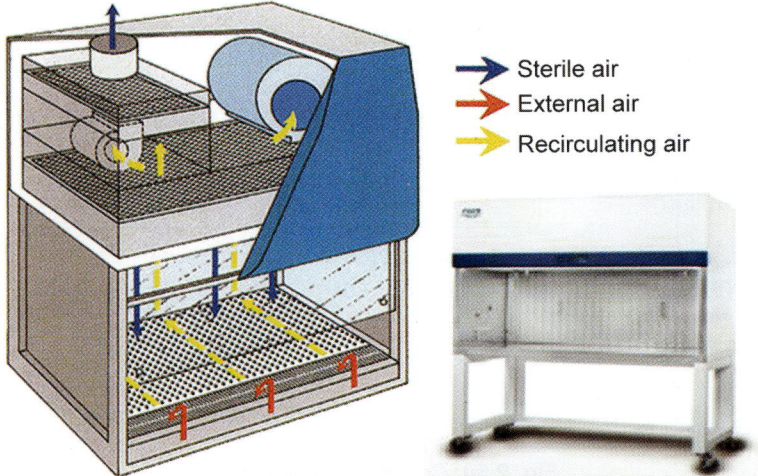

Fig. 4.7: Vertical laminar airflow cabinet

1 Introduction to Scope of Microbiology

I. Introduction to Microbiology
II. Definitions
III. Classification of Microorganisms
IV. The Place of Microorganisms in the Living World
    E. H. Haeckel's Kingdom Protista
    Prokaryotic and Eukaryotic Protists
    Whittaker's Five Kingdom Concept
V. Spontaneous Generation of Organisms
VI. Historical Background of Microbiology
    Edward Jenner (1749–1823)
    John Tyndall (1820–1893)
    Louis Pasteur (1822–1895)
    Pasteur and Diseases
    Robert Koch (1843–1910)
VII. Types of Microorganisms
    Bacteria
    Archaea
    Fungi
    Protozoa
    Algae
    Viruses
    Multicellular Animal Parasites
VIII. Application and Scope of Microbiology
IX. Future of Microbiology
    Important Study Question

I. INTRODUCTION TO MICROBIOLOGY

India can take pride that it contributes to the development of ancient microbiology in the form of septic tanks in *Mohenjo-daro* and *Harappa* regions (3000 B.C.). But *Leeuwenhoek* (1677) could see the microbes in simple (one lens) microscope and established the existence of microbes. *Leeuwenhoek*, a cloth merchant in Delft, Holland spend much of his time in grinding tiny lenses of high magnification (300X or so).

Golden era of microbiology started with the work of *Louis Pasteur* (France) and *Robert Koch* (Germany). *Louis Pasteur* (1822–1895) invented that boiled medium could remain clear in a "Swan-neck" flask, which is open to the air through a sinuous horizontal tube in which dust particle will be settled as air re-entered the cooling vessel.

II. DEFINITIONS

Microbiology: It is defined as the biological science which deals with the study of microorganisms. This includes viruses, bacteria, fungi, algae and protozoa.

Microorganism/Microbes/Germs: They are defined as living organisms which are very small, microscopic in size that cannot be seen with the human necked eye.

III. CLASSIFICATION OF MICROORGANISMS

Before the existence of the microbes was known, all the organisms were grouped into either the animal kingdom or the plant kingdom. When microscopic organisms with characteristics of animals or plants were discovered, a new system of classification was required. Still biologists could not agree on the criteria for classifying the new organism they were seeing until the late 1970s. In 1987, *Carl Woese* divided a system of classification based on the cellular organization of the organisms. It groups all organisms in three domains as follows:

1. Bacteria (cell walls consist of a protein-carbohydrate complex called peptidoglycan)
2. Archaea (cell walls, if present, lack peptidoglycan)
3. Eukarya, which includes the following:
   - Protists (slime molds, protozoa and algae)
   - Fungi (unicellular *yeasts*, multicellular *molds* and *mushrooms*)

- Plants (includes *mosses, ferns, conifers,* and *flowering plants*)
- Animals (includes *sponges, worms,* insects and vertebrates)

IV. THE PLACE OF MICROORGANISMS IN THE LIVING WORLD

In biology as in any other field, classification means the orderly arrangement of units under study into groups of larger units. Present day classification in biology was established by the work of *Carolus Linnaeus* (1701–1778), a Swedish botanist. His books on the classification of plants and animals are considered to be beginning of modern botanical and zoological nomenclature, a system of naming plants and animals. Nomenclature in microbiology, which came much later, was based on the principles established for the plant and animal kingdoms.

Until the 18th century, all the living organisms including microorganisms were classified in the classification of living organisms placed all microorganisms into one of two kingdoms, plant and animal. As previously stated, in microbiology we study some organisms that are predominantly plant like and others that are animal like, also some that share characteristics common to both plants and animals. There are organisms that do not fall naturally into either the plant or animal kingdom, hence new kingdoms were proposed to be established to include those organisms which typically are neither plants nor animals.

E. H. Haeckel's Kingdom Protista

One of the earliest of these proposals was made in 1866 by a German zoologist *E.H.Haeckel*. He suggested that a third kingdom protista, be formed to include those unicellular microorganisms that are typically neither plants nor animal.

These organisms, the protists, include bacteria, algae, fungi and protozoa viruses are not cellular organisms and therefore are not classified as *protists*. Bacteria are referred as lower protists; the others, algae, fungi and protozoa, are called higher protists.

Prokaryotic and Eukaryotic Protists

Hackel's kingdom protista left some questions unanswered. For example, what criteria could be used to distinguish a *bacterium* from *yeast* or certain microscopic algae?

Satisfactory criteria were unavailable until late in the 1940s when more definitive observation of internal cell structure was made possible with the aid of the powerful magnification provided by electron microscopy. It was discovered that in some cells, for example, typical bacteria, the nuclear substances was not enclosed by a nuclear membrane. In other cells, such as typical algae and fungi, the nucleus was enclosed in a membrane. The discovery that the absence of membrane bound internal structures in one group of protists (bacteria) and the presence of membrane bound structure in others (algae, fungi, and protozoa) was a discovery of fundamental significance. Further research has revealed additional differences in the internal structure of these cells.

Whittaker's Five Kingdom Concept

A more recent and comprehensive system of classification, the five kingdom system, was proposed by *R.H.Whittaker* (1969). This system of classification, shown in Fig. 1.1, is based on three levels of cellular organization which evolves to accommodate three principal modes of nutrition, i.e. photosynthesis, absorption and ingestion.

The prokaryotes are included in the kingdom *monera*; they lack the ingestive mode of nutrition. Unicellular eukaryotic microorganisms are placed in the kingdom protista; all three nutritional types are represented here. In fact, as shown in Fig. 1.1, the nutritional modes are continuous. The mode of nutrition of the *microalgae* is photosynthetic, the mode of nutrition of protozoa is ingestive, and the mode of nutrition in some other protists is adsorptive, with some overlap to the photosynthetic and ingestive modes.

The multicellular and multinucleate eukaryotic organisms are found in the kingdoms *plantae* (multicellular green plants and higher algae), kingdom *animalia* (multicellular animals) and kingdom fungi (multinucleate higher fungi). Their diversified nutritional modes lead to a more diversified cellular organization. Microorganism are found in three of the five kingdoms; monera (bacteria and *cyanobacteria*), protista (*microalgae* and *protozoa*) and fungi (*yeasts* and *molds*).

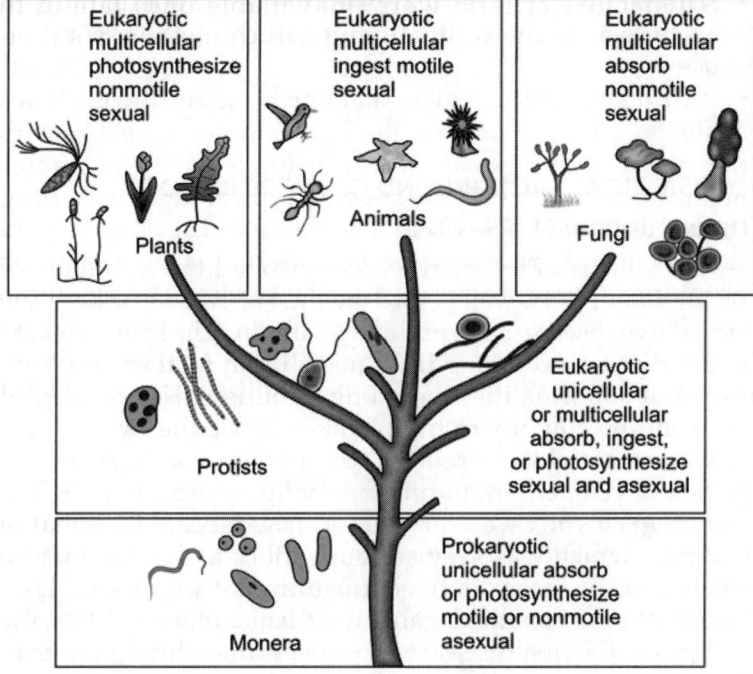

Fig. 1.1: Schematic representation of Whittaker's five kingdom theory

V. SPONTANEOUS GENERATION OF ORGANISMS

The theory of spontaneous generation states that "non-living objects give rise to living organism". That is why it is believed that microbes arise automatically in decomposing organic matter.

- In the 17th century *Francesco Redi* had seen the *maggots* in decomposing meat which was dependent on decomposition of Flies' eggs.
- *T. Needham* (1748) experienced the organisms appeared from the decomposition of the vegetables and meat.
- Later *Spallanzani* (1729–1799) introduced the use of sterile culture media, i.e. the infusion of meat would remain clear for indefinite period of time if it is boiled and properly sealed.
- *Schwann* (1837) and *Liebig* (1839) did experiments of alcoholic fermentation and putrefaction.

- *Schroder* and *Von Dusch* applied the use of cotton plug, to exclude airborne contaminants which method is still in use.
- *Pasteur* gave the statement that 'life is a germ and germ is a life'.

VI. HISTORICAL BACKGROUND OF MICROBIOLOGY

Edward Jenner (1749-1823)

He was a British Physician who developed the technique of vaccination in 1795, well before the time of *Pasteur* or *Koch*. He studied two diseases: cowpox and smallpox. The smallpox was deadly disease occurring in humans often fatal or resulting in several abnormalities including blindness. He transferred pus from the cowpox to human skin. Since the two disease organisms are closely related, the person vaccinated with cowpox developed, immunity to smallpox virus as well. The reaction to cowpox was very minor/insignificant than that of smallpox, which was very serious. Till date the vaccination developed by *Jenner* is used for elimination of smallpox disease. World Health Organization has announced that the smallpox is the first disease to become extinct through human efforts.

John Tyndall (1820-1893)

It was not universally proved that boiling could kill all microorganisms in a broth. *John Tyndall* was an English Physicist who confirmed the results of *Pasteur's* experiments. He demonstrated that heating might not damage all the microbes present in the heated material. The difference is due to the capacity of bacteria to exist in two forms like:

1. A heat liable form, likely to be killed by the exposure to heat that was destroyed by the exposures of elevated temperatures and
2. The heat resistance form that could survive at such high temperatures. According to him an intermitted heating of a solution can eliminate viable microorganisms and thus sterilize solutions, which completely eliminate living microbes from them. This validates *Pasteur's* negation of spontaneous generation. Repeated heating on successive days is known as *tyndallization*. The alternate heating

(121°C) water under pressure 15 ponds/sq inch can sterilize the solution.

Louis Pasteur: A Founding Father: (1822–1895)

Louis Pasteur was one of the scientists of his day. His achievements served as stepping stones for others. He succeeded in defining the theory of spontaneous generation. He established that living microorganisms are responsible for the chemical changes that occur during fermentation. He confirmed that certain microbes were directly responsible for the formation of different types of molecule as acetic acid and lactic acid. He was trained as a chemist. He was appointed as a Dean of Science Faculty at University of Lille (1854). A local industrialist requested him to solve the problem of alcohol souring produced by him. He solved the problem and he became microbiologist from a chemist. He collected the samples from the souring alcohol and observed under microscope. He found that sour wine vats contain rod shaped organisms together with budding yeasts cells. He explained that these two organisms determine the course of the chemical processes that results in different fermentations. The *yeasts* were responsible for the production of alcohol and the rod shaped bacteria produce lactic acid, which cause souring of wine.

In 1857, *Pasteur* demonstrated that souring of milk is due to the action of microorganisms and in 1860 he demonstrated that heating could be used to kill microorganisms in wine and beer. The process was named after him as pasteurization (heating moderate temperatures to reduce the number of living microorganisms). He reported on organized bodies, which exist in the atmosphere, an examination of the doctrine of spontaneous generation. *Pasteur* was of the opinion that when liquids are subjected to boiling they remain sterile, that is, free from all kinds of living microorganisms; as long as micro-organisms in the air are not allowed contaminating the liquid.

Pasteur and Diseases

He used gooseneck flask for studies. It is a long curved flask. He kept the sterile fermentable substrate in this flask, open into the air and demonstrated that fermentation did not occurred. The special shape of the flask restricted the entry of airborne

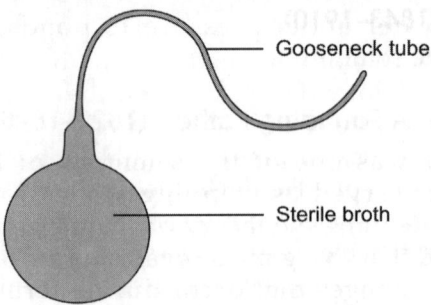

Fig. 1.2: Gooseneck flask

microorganism from entering the liquid; and the air could not enter the flask. He also demonstrated the presence of bacteria in the air.

He found that airborne organisms could be kept out of sterile materials by plugging the tops with sterile cotton and still have air circulation in the bottle. *Pasteur* was influenced by the work of *Robert Koch* who demonstrated that the bacterium cause anthrax in cattle. The excitement generated by *Koch* encouraged *Pasteur* to work on the anthrax disease. *Pasteur* demonstrated that prevention of anthrax in cattle by injecting healthy animals with live anthrax bacteria that had been specially treated to reduce their disease causing abilities. His success with anthrax led him to investigate hydrophobia or rabies.

Louis Pasteur made several discoveries in the fields of microbiology. The important are as follows:

1. He could be able to separate two types' tartaric acid crystals with the help of microscope.
2. The fermentation is a vital chemical process, which is brought about by the activity of microorganisms like *yeast* and bacteria, which do not cause disease.
3. Presence of microorganisms in air.
4. He introduced the terms anaerobic and aerobic. He discovered aerobic life
5. Immunization of sheep against anthrax.

Louis Pasteur is known to the world as one of the great scientist. He is credited with starting microbiologists dawn a path of research in the area of preventive medicine and immunology. In the year 1888, *Pasteur* laid the foundation of Pasteur Institute in Paris.

Robert Koch (1843-1910)

He was German Doctor who made several discoveries in the fields of microbiology. He discovered that bacteria can be isolated and can cause diseases which he proved while working with anthrax disease of animals. He gave the final proof of these concepts. He developed the *Koch's* postulates, which means that a specific microorganism is responsible for the cause of specific disease. He developed the technique of pure culture. He also discovered the bacterium that caused anthrax in cattle and demonstrated the progression of the disease. He isolated and identified various kinds of micro-organisms specially bacteria. So he is regarded as the first true bacteriologist. He is also known as founder of medical microbiology, bacteriology and virology. He was a physician and was practicing as a Doctor in small German town. He found anthrax disease begins with symptoms similar to a cold and causes itching skin, blisters or vesicles form which later turn black and swell. The bacteria may move in to the blood and cause fever. *Koch* isolated the bacterium that caused anthrax. He injected laboratory animal with the anthrax bacteria which was detected in the blood of dead sheep. He then performed autopsies and recorded how the same symptoms appear regularly. He injected mice with a sawdust of wood containing endospores and found that the mice develops anthrax symptoms. On observing blood samples, several thread like bacteria were present in it. He also studied that anthrax bacterium in frogs and horses and demonstrated that how the disease causing microbe became concentrated in the lymph sacs and spleen. *Koch's* postulates state as follows:

1. A particular organism can always be found in association with a particular disease, but not in healthy individual.
2. The organism can be grown in the laboratory itself.
3. The pure microbial culture will produce the same disease when placed back into a new susceptible animal.
4. It is possible to recover the organism from the sick animal and grow them in pure culture.

On the above basis it was concluded by the microbiologists that a particular microbe is in fact the cause of particular disease. *Koch* isolated the bacillus responsible for causing *tuberculosis*. He confirmed the theory of *John Snow* that water is the important cause for the transmission of disease. *Koch* was appointed to the University of Berlin (1885) and was made Director of Institute of Infectious Diseases in 1890. He continued his work on tuberculosis and was rewarded for this work with the Nobel Prize in 1905.

VII. TYPES OF MICROORGANISMS

Bacteria

Bacteria or *bacterium* are relatively simple, single celled/ unicellular organism. Bacterial cell are called prokaryotes because their genetic material is not enclosed in a special nuclear membrane. Bacterial cell generally appears in the one of several shapes. *Bacillus* (rod-like), *Coccus* (spherical or ovoid) and *Spiral* (cork screw or curved) are most common shapes but some bacteria are also in star shaped, coma shaped or square shaped. Individual bacteria may form pairs, chains, clusters or other groupings. These formations are usually characteristic of a particular genus or species of bacteria. Bacteria are enclosed in the cell walls which are largely composed of carbohydrate and protein complex called *peptidoglycan*. Bacteria generally reproduce by dividing into two equal cells; this process is called binary fission. For nutrition, most bacteria use organic chemicals, which in nature can be derived from either dead or living organisms. Some bacteria can manufacture their own food by photosynthesis and some can derive nutrition from inorganic substances. Many bacteria can swim by using moving appendages called flagella.

Archaea

It consist of prokaryotic cells like bacteria but they have cell walls which lacks peptidoglycan. Archaea are often found in extreme environment and are divided into three main groups. The *methanogens* produce methane as a waste product from respiration. The extreme *halophiles* live in extremely salty environments such as the Great Salt Lake and the Dead Sea. The extreme *thermophiles* live in hot sulfurous water such as hot springs at Yellowstone national park. *Archaea* are not known to cause disease in humans.

Fungi

Fungi are eukaryotes organism whose cells have a distinct nucleus containing the cell's genetic material (DNA), surrounded by a special envelope called nuclear membrane. Organisms may be unicellular or multicellular. Large multicellular fungi, such as *mushroom* may look somewhat like plants but they cannot carry out photosynthesis like other plants.

True fungi have cell walls composed of substance called chitin. The unicellular forms of fungi, *yeasts* are oval microorganisms that are larger than bacteria. The most typical fungi are *molds*. *Molds* form visible masses called *mycelia*, which are composed of long filaments that branch and intertwined. The cottony growths sometimes found on bread and fruit are *mold mycelia*.

Fungi can reproduce sexually or asexually. It produces the hydrolytic enzymes which digest the organic matter and convert to the soluble form. They obtain nourishment by absorbing solutions of digested organic material from their environment whether soil, sea water, fresh water or an animal or plant host. Organisms called *slime molds* have characteristics of both fungi and amoebas.

Protozoa

Protozoa or protozoans are unicellular, eukaryotic microbes. Protozoa move by pseudo pods (false feet), flagella or cilia. *Amoebas* move by using extensions of their cytoplasm called pseudo pods. Other protozoa have long flagella or numerous shorter appendages for locomotion called cilia. Protozoa have a variety of shapes and live either as free entities or as parasite (derives nutrients from living hosts) that absorb or ingest organic compounds from their environment. Protozoa can reproduce sexually or asexually.

Algae

Algae are photosynthetic eukaryotes with a wide variety of shapes and both sexual and asexual reproductive forms. The algae of interest to microbiologists are usually unicellular. The cell walls of many algae, like those of plants, are composed of a carbohydrate called cellulose. The algae are abundant in fresh and salt water, in soil and in association with plants. As photo synthesizers, algae need light, water, and carbon dioxide for food production and growth, they do not generally require organic compound from the environment. As a result of photosynthesis, algae produce oxygen and carbohydrates that are then utilized by other organisms, including animals. Thus, they play an important role in the balance of nature.

Viruses

Viruses are very different from the other microbial groups mentioned above. They are so small that most can be seen only with an electron microscope, and they are acellular (not cellular). Structurally very simple, a virus particle contains a core made of only one type of nucleic acid, either DNA or RNA. This core is surrounded by a protein coat. Sometimes the coat is encased by an additional layer, a lipid membrane called an envelope. All living cells have RNA and DNA, which can carry out chemical reactions and can reproduce as self-sufficient units.

Virus can reproduce only by using the cellular machinery of the other organisms. Thus on the one hand viruses are considered to be living when they multiply within the host cells they infect. In this sense, viruses are parasites to other forms of life. On the other hand, viruses are not considered to be living because outside of living hosts they are inert. Thus viruses can be considered as connecting link between nonliving and living organisms.

Multicellular Animal Parasites

Although multicellular animal parasites are not strictly microorganisms, they are of medical importance. The two major groups of parasitic worms are the *flatworms* and the *round worms*, collectively called *helminths*. During some stages of their life cycle, *helminths* are microscopic in size. Laboratory identification of these organisms included many of the same techniques used for the identification of microbes.

VIII. APPLICATION AND SCOPE OF MICROBIOLOGY

The microorganisms influence the man in several ways. The microorganisms are ubiquitous in our environment, i.e. they are found in soil, mud, water, air, in animals, plants, food products dead wood, cloths, jams, shoes, optical instruments, nails, skin, even in the space and at Antarctica.

The diversity of their activity varies from causing disease in human and other animals and plants to the production of various useful products, recovery of metals, increasing the soil fertility and the deterioration of aeroplanes.

The chief fields of microbiology are described below

1. Microbiology in food and dairy industries: Food microbiology involves the study of microbes which provide food due to their high protein value (e.g. *yeast)* and also the microbes which uses our food supply as a source of nutrient, for their growth and result in deterioration of the food.

Many special *molds* are useful in the manufacture of certain foods and ingredients of the foods. Some cheese is *mold* ripened. *Molds* are also used in production of oriental foods, e.g. soya sauce and miso. *Molds* are involved in making enzymes such as amylase for bread making, citric acid for making soft drinks, etc. Some *molds* are harmful and some produce toxic metabolites.

Yeast may also be useful or harmful in food, *yeast* fermentations are used in manufacture of foods such as bread, beer, wines, vinegar and surface ripened cheese. *Yeast* is undesirable when they spoil fruit juices, syrups, molasses, jam, pickles, wine, beer and other foods.

2. In the production of industrial products: Enzymes, amino acids, vitamins, antibiotics, organic acids and alcohols are commercially produced by microorganisms.

Some of these products are used by microbes during their growth. They are called primary microbial products or primary metabolites, e.g. enzymes, amino acids and vitamins. Some of these products are not used by the cell for their growths are called as secondary microbial products or secondary metabolites, e.g. antibiotics, alcohol and organic acids.

Enzyme lipases are used in detergents such as Surf. Enzyme proteases are also used in detergents and also in leather and food industries. Various small quantities of other enzymes of microbial origin such as asparaginase is used against leukemia (blood cancer), lymphomas (cancer) which act upon high percentage of amino acid aspargin that are present in cancer cells. Microbes produce some important amino acids such as glutamic acid, lysine and methionine. The citric acid, a Krebs's cycle (TCA cycle) intermediate is mainly produced by *Aspergillus niger*.

3. In genetic engineering and biotechnology: Molecular technique which is used for manipulating the genetic information is called genetic engineering and the use of such genetically engineered microbes in industrial processes are called biotechnology. Microorganisms now a day are used to produce the mammalian proteins such as insulin and human growth factor, to make vaccines from microbial and viral genes and to induce the new strains of microbes. Interferons are produced in animal cells by viral infectants. These are also used in testing of interleukins.

By the use of genetic engineering and biotechnology, it is possible to have production of viral, bacterial and protozoan antigen for protecting human against dysentery, typhoid, cholera, etc. It is also possible to produce viral vaccines against flu or influenza, chickenpox and human immunodeficiency, e.g. viral vaccines that consist of cloned polypeptide antigens are produced by genetic engineering to prevent foot, mouth disease and hepatitis B.

Microorganisms can make some of the important vitamins such as vitamin B_{12}, which cannot be made by human body. Riboflavin (Vit. B_2) is produced by *yeast Ashbya gossypii*. Antibiotics such as β-lactum are used in various treatment purposes. Penicillin is the good choice for the treatment of gonococcal, treponemal and streptococcal infection. Transformants producing VP_3 protein were used to make vaccines that protect the foot and mouth disease in animals. In future, some more new vaccines would be required for check of protozoan disease that affects the people.

4. In environmental microbiology: Microbes are present everywhere, i.e. in soil, water, and air. They are also present in deep inside the earth such as sea vents. Microbes require oxygen, carbon, nitrogen, sulphur and phosphorus like components as nutrients for their growth, which are directly and easily available to all the microbes, e.g. water is a product of aerobic processes, so, again remains available for photosynthesis for microbes.

Viruses that infect living cells can create the water pollution problem. Again, *plant virus* and *algae virus* can prevent the development of the host. So, it is suggested that excessive growth of *blue green algae* can be controlled by seeding with specific viruses. Similarly, *bacterial viruses (bacteriophage)* may help in controlling the size of bacterial population through the lysis of susceptible group. The *bacteriophage* play role in destruction of bacteria which are pathogenic to man and present in fecal pollution, but on the other hand, bacteria play a role to exploit the wide range of environmental opportunities. Complex microbial population plays an important role in self-purification and they will dominate the ecology of treatment plants. Some organic molecules present in industrial effluents are readily decomposed by variety of microorganisms.

5. Microbes and medical microbiology: Microbes cause infections in humans and animals and thus results in diseases among them. The control of infectious disease is the greatest achievement of medical science, e.g. vaccination reduces the incidence of several epidemic diseases. Living cells infected with viruses produce viral proteins (glycoproteins) which are called as interferon. These interferons have a broad spectrum of antiviral action. Interferon has a number of biological effects and also inhibits the parasitic infections caused by *chlamydia, rickettsiae,* protozoa and bacteria. Antibiotics derived from various *fungi,* streptomyces are extensively used to control the diseases in human and animals.

6. Development of fermentation models: Microbes help in fermentation process. By using mathematical models, it is possible to understand the fermentation process. The use of model can also help in development of better control strategies for fermentation.

7. Microbes in agriculture: Some of the important areas where the different groups of microorganisms participate in agriculture are organic composting, increasing soil fertility, reclamation of alkaline user land, use as biofertilizer and microbial pesticides.

In complete and artificially composting, the organic matter is mixed with microbial population in moist, warm and aerobic conditions. It also helps in preparation and application of organic anaerobic environment. The microbial conversion of the complex organic materials favors built up of the nutrient rich compost, within the short span. This organic compost is the storehouse of major plant nutrient and micronutrients. Microbiological conversion of organic materials into methane gas through anaerobic digestion has been quite successful in recent years. The productivity of leguminous crops largely depends on an efficient management of eco-system which involves specific rhizobial association. The association of *rhizobia* and other category of bacteria offer an advantage that the molecular nitrogen is converted into assimilable form of ammonia and thus help the crops to grow purely on the biological sources of nitrogen. Certain plant *pathogenic fungi* causing disease (such as charcoal rot, collar rot, damping off will, etc.) in plants can be checked by using various bacteria (like *Burkholderia cepacia* syn. *Pseudomonas cepacia* and *P. fluorescens*) and fungi (like *Gliocladium virens* and *Trichoderma harzianum*). There are several laboratories involved in research on microbial insecticides. Large scale efforts are required in controlling agricultural pests, nematodes and mosquitoes through microbial manipulations.

8. Microbes in bio-terrorism: Bio-terrorism means the deliberate release of disease causing microorganisms which are intended to kill large number of people and panic many more. In short, the microorganisms are used as weapons of mass destruction.

Some of these microorganisms cause smallpox, plague and cholera but the anthrax, caused by *Bacillus anthracis* can kill millions. When *anthrax spores* enters the body, it grows rapidly and produce anthrax toxin in the body which kills the cells of the immune system. It can occur as skin anthrax, intestinal anthrax and inhalation anthrax. Another infectious agent is *Yersinia pestis*, transmitted by the infected rat flea to human beings and animals and cause plague. A large number of microorganisms including large number of bacteria (*Bacilus anthracis, Brucella abortus, Yersinia pestis*, etc.) and viruses (*Crimean congo, Hemorrhagic fever virus, Ebola virus, Lassa fever virus, Variola* (smallpox), *major virus*, etc.) can create terror to both human and animals. Though during 20th century, about 300 million people died due to smallpox. This virus spread from person to person, usually by droplet infection. There is no natural resistance to smallpox except prior vaccination.

9. *Computer application:* Computer application in microbiology is not yet as widespread as in the chemical industry but still sensor by computer for use of sterile system is advantageous. Computer can serve a variety of function is in fermentation process control and analysis. Computers are used in scale up, to store the parameters, evaluate the fermentation parameters and to measure the effect of individual parameters on the behaviors of cultures. Online fermentation control is widely used in the production scale in many companies.

IX. FUTURE OF MICROBIOLOGY

Microbiology has great practical significance. It has a clearer mission than other scientific disciplines. Medical biology, public health microbiology, and immunology will continue to be areas of intense research. New infectious diseases are continuously arising and old diseases are once again becoming widespread and destructive. AIDS, SARS, hemorrhagic fevers and tuberculosis are excellent examples of new diseases. Microbiologists will have to respond to these threats, many of them presently unknown. They will also need to find the ways to stop the spread of established infectious diseases and also the spread of multiple antibiotic resistances, which can render a pathogen resistant to current medical treatment. Microbiologists are also required to create new drugs and vaccines to study the association between infectious agents and chronic disease and to further understanding of host defenses and how pathogens interact with host cells. It may be necessary to use techniques in molecular biology and recombinant DNA technology to solve many of these problems.

Industrial microbiology and environmental microbiology also face many challenges and opportunities. Microorganisms are increasingly important in industry and environmental control. For example, microorganisms can serve as sources of high quality food and other practical products such as enzymes for industrial applications. They may also be used to degrade pollutants and toxic wastes and as vectors to treat diseases and enhance agricultural productivity. There is also a continuing need to protect food and crops from microbial damage. The discovery of new and unusual microorganisms may lead to further advances in the development of new antimicrobial agents, industrial processes and bioremediation.

Another area of increasing interest to microbial ecologists is biofilms. They are not only of interest to microbial ecologists; they can form on human tissues, on indwelling catheters, and on the manmade medical devices. The fields of genomics and proteomics have and will continue to have a tremendous impact on microbiology. The genomes of many microorganisms have already been sequenced and many more will be determined in the coming years. These sequences are ideal for learning how the genome is related to cell structure and function and for providing insights into fundamental questions in biology, such as how complex cellular structures develop and how cells communicate with one another and respond to the environment. The pace of the new discoveries and developments is very rapid and the field of microbiology and biotechnology will provide major contribution to it.

IMPORTANT STUDY QUESTIONS

1. Define pharmaceutical microbiology. Describe its scope in brief. (Dec 2010, Dec 2011, June 2011)
2. Describe contribution of 'Louis Pasteur' in microbiology. (Dec 2010)
3. Define microbiology and give its applications.
4. What is Whittaker's five kingdom concept?
5. Give historical importance of Robert Koch.
6. Write a note on need of microbiology in future development.

2
General Microbiology

I. Microscopy
  A. Light Microscopy
    1. Bright Field Microscope
    2. Dark Field Microscope
    3. Phase Contrast Microscope
    4. Differential Interference Contrast (DIC) Microscope
    5. Fluorescence Microscope
    6. Confocal Microscope
  B. Electron Microscopy
    1. Transmission Electron Microscope
    2. Scanning Electron Microscope
  C. Scanned Probe Microscopy
    1. Scanning Tunneling Microscopy (STM)
    2. Atomic Force Microscopy (AFM)
II. Staining Technique
  A. Definition
  B. Importance of Staining
  C. Theories of Staining
  D. Classification of Stains
  E. Types of Staining
    1. Simple Staining
    2. Differential Staining Technique
    3. Special Staining
III. Classification and Taxonomy
  A. Major Characteristics Used in Classification
  B. General Methods Used in Classification of Microorganism
  C. Prokaryotic and Eukaryotic Cells
IV. Bacteria
  A. General Characteristics of Bacteria
  B. Classification of Bacteria

V. Actinomycetes

    A. General Characteristics of Actinomycetes

    B. Examples of Actinomycetes

VI. Fungi

VII. Rickettsia

VIII. Spirochetes

IX. Protozoa

X. Structure of Bacterial Cell

XI. Nutritional Requirements of Bacteria

    A. Nutrition Required for the Growth

    B. Nutrient Media Required for the Growth

    C. Physical Condition Required for the Nutrition and Growth

XII. Cultivation of Bacteria

XIII. Growth Cycle of Bacteria

XIV. Types of Growth

    1. Synchronous Growth

    2. Diauxic Growth

    3. Continuous Growth

XV. Reproduction of Bacteria

XVI. Isolation of Bacteria

XVII. Viruses

    A. General Characteristics of Viruses

    B. Classification of Virus

XVIII. Structure of Viruses

XIX. Bacteriophage

XX. Nutritional Requirement of Virus

XXI. Cultivation of Viruses

    A. Cultivation of Animal Virus

    B. Cultivation of Bacteriophages (Bacterial Virus)

    C. Cultivation of Plant Viruses

XXII. Multiplication of Bacterial Virus (Bacteriophage)/Life Cycle of Bacteriophages

XXIII. Isolation and Identification of Viruses

I. MICROSCOPY

Microscope is an optical instrument consisting of a lens or combination of lenses used for making enlarged or magnified images of minute objects such as microbes which cannot be seen by unaided (necked) eye. The science that deals with all the aspects of microscope is called *Microscopy*.

The objective of microscopy is to magnify the image, to maximize resolution and to get the sufficient contrast to distinguish the different components of microorganisms. Microscopy can be classified as follows:

1. **Depending on the number of lenses**
   a. Simple microscope which contains single lens
   b. Compound microscope which contains two lenses or more
2. **Depending on the number of eyepiece**
   a. Monocular microscope that contains single eyepiece.
   b. Binocular microscope which contains two eyepieces.
3. **Depending on the source**
   a. Light or optical microscope which uses optical lenses and visible light
   b. Electron microscope which uses electromagnetic lenses and electron beam

Numerical aperture: Consider the most divergent ray passing through the objective, then θ is the angle between the axis of the lens system and the most divergent ray (Fig. 2.1).

Based on θ, the numerical aperture $= n \sin \theta$, where, $n =$ refractive index of the medium.

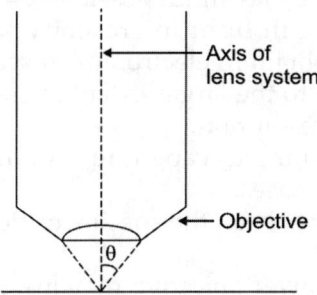

Fig. 2.1: Numerical aperture

"Numerical aperture is the sin value of the half aperture angle multiplied by the refractive index n of the medium, filling the space between the front lens and the cover slip". Resolution power is directly proportional to numerical aperture. Numerical aperture is the characteristics of a lens system.

Resolution power: Microscope must produce a clear image along with the magnified image. The magnification efficiency of the compound microscope is given by its resolution power. Resolution is the ability of a lens to separate or distinguish between small objects that are close together.

Resolution is the function of the wavelength of light used and numerical aperture of the lens system.

$$d(\mu m) = \frac{0.5\lambda}{\eta \sin \theta}$$

d = minimum distance between two objects that can be separate distinctly.

λ = wavelength

As d becomes smaller, the resolution increases, e.g. Numerical aperture = 1.25; λ_{max} = 530 nm (blue green light)

Then $\qquad d = \dfrac{0.5 \times 530}{1.25} = 212$ nm $= 0.2$ μm

Numerical aperture = 1.00; λ_{max} = 0.005 nm (wavelength of electron)

$$d = \frac{0.5 \times 0.005}{1.00} = 0.0025 \text{ nm}$$

As seen above the maximum possible resolution that can be obtained is 0.2 μm in light microscopy while 2×10^{-6} μm resolution can be obtain in electron microscopy. Thus, we can magnify the image to the larger extent in electron microscopy because of higher resolution.

Similarly, if the numerical aperture of the objective increases, then resolution increases.

As the distance between the specimens decreases, the angle θ increase (Fig. 2.2).

So, the higher power objective remains, much more closes to the specimen. The maximum angle θ can be close to 90 and

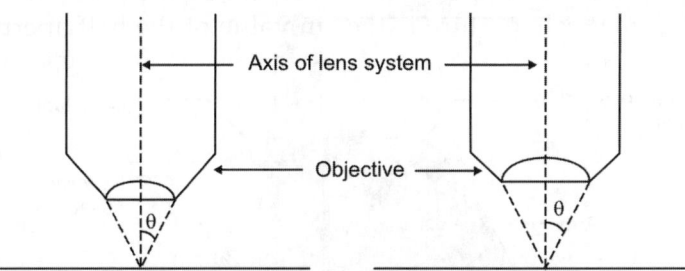

Fig. 2.2: Correlation between numerical aperture and resolution

Sin 90 is 1.00. The refractive index of air is 1.0. So no lens working in air can have numerical aperture greater than 1.00.

The only way to raise the numerical aperture above 1.00 is to increase the refractive index by using immersion oil.

Cedarwood oil is used as immersion oil as it has same refractive index as of glass that is 1.5. Thus, NA greater than 1 can be obtained.

Many light rays do not enter the objective due to reflection and refraction when they pass from glass cover slip and air. If air is replaced with cedarwood oil, there will be no reflection and refraction taking place and most light rays from specimen are visualized. Numerical aperture and resolution increases.

A. Light Microscopy

The microscope which uses the light as a source of illumination is called light microscopy.

The different types of light microscopes are as follows:

1. Bright Field Microscope
2. Dark Field Microscope
3. Phase Contrast Microscope
4. Differential Interference Contrast (DIC) Microscope
5. Fluorescence Microscope
6. Confocal Microscope

1. Bright Field Microscope

The microscope that produced dark image against the bright background is known as bright field microscope. The most widely used bright field microscope is the *compound microscope* (Fig. 2.3).

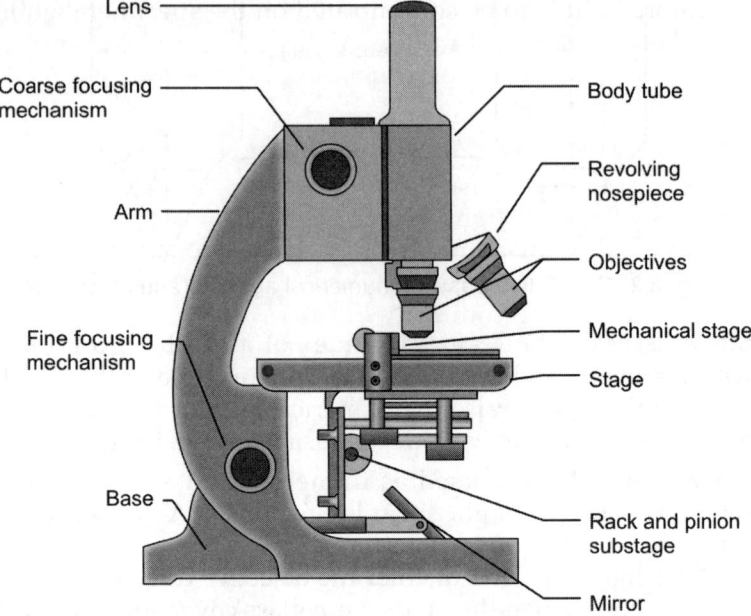

Lens

Coarse focusing mechanism

Body tube

Revolving nosepiece

Arm

Objectives

Mechanical stage

Fine focusing mechanism

Stage

Base

Rack and pinion substage

Mirror

Fig. 2.3: Compound microscope

Principle

The mirror reflects the light rays towards the condenser. The condenser forms the cone of light from the reflected rays. This cone of light strikes on an object. The light ray picks up the details of the object and enters in the objective. The objective produces an enlarged, real and inverted primary image. The primary image forms at upper part of body tube. The eyepiece further magnifies the primary image with the help of field lens. The function of the field lens is to collect the diverging rays of primary image and forms a virtual image. Thus, image seen by retina of eye is a virtual image, which is formed by eyepiece (Fig. 2.3).

Construction and working

1. *Base:* It supports and stabilizes the microscope.
2. *Illuminator (source of light):* The source of light for this type of microscope may be a simple mirror. A concave mirror is used if condenser is not equipped in the microscope or

more light is to be concentrated on the specimen, while a plane surface mirror is used if the condenser is equipped in the microscope. In some microscopes an in-built illuminator (lamp) is equipped.

3. *Illumination*

   a. *Critical type:* It is described by Abbe and Nelson. In this system, the light source, such as sun light through a window or an open lamp flame is placed before the microscope mirror. Any structure or irregularity of the source is seen directly in the field of view. It creates a problem to some extent during examination of the specimen.

   b. *Kochler's type:* It is prepared by *Dr. August Kochler.* The *Kochler* form of illumination is mostly used today. Here, the parallel rays of light is generated by a tungsten filament lamp are used for the illumination of the specimen. It eliminates the disadvantages of the first method, i.e. it insures a full and evenly illuminated field of view.

4. *Mechanical stage:* It is the platform on which the specimen to be viewed is placed. Some stages have clips to hold the glass slide in place and other stages have a mechanical stage, which make it possible to move the glass slide across the stage in both the direction, horizontal and vertical.

5. *Focus adjustment knobs:* There are two focus adjustment knobs, a coarse adjustment and a fine adjustment. They are used to move the body tubes/stage relative to the objectives and ocular which makes it possible to focus the image. Nowaday, in most modern microscopes, the fine focus knob is built into the coarse focus knob.

6. *Body tube:* It holds ocular and objective lenses. It provides the sufficient space for image formation

7. *Nosepiece:* It is the base in which objectives are fixed. Simply rotating the nosepiece can rotate each objective in to place.

8. *Lenses*

   a. *Eyepiece:* It is also referred as ocular. It is the first lens system of a microscope. It stands at the top of the microscope. In the microscope, the ocular is capable of 10X magnifications. In recent, eyepieces of 5X, 15X and 20X magnification potential are also available.

Function: To make a magnified virtual image of specimen.

b. *Objective lenses:* It is the second lens system of the microscope. These are mounted on a nosepiece and can be rotated into the place. There are usually three or more objective lenses on the microscope. The objective lenses are generally equipped with microscope having a low power, high power and oil immersion lens and magnification of 10X, 45X and 100X respectively.

Function: To make magnified real.

c. *Condenser:* It is the third lens system of microscope. It is located below the stage. It is responsible for the focusing of light on the specimen. There are several various types of condensers depending upon the type of microscopy to be employed.

Function: It makes sufficient cone of light.

9. *Iris diaphragm:* It is equipped with condenser. It controls the intensity of light entering the condenser and by that it controls the amount of light intensity. Lever is equipped with it to adjust the light intensity. Blue color filter is also equipped below the condenser.

2. Dark Field Microscope

The microscope that forms bright image against dark background is called as dark field microscope.

Principle

It is used for examination of live microorganisms which are invisible in the ordinary light microscope or which cannot be stained by standard methods or which can be distorted by staining so that its characteristics cannot be identified. A dark field microscope uses a dark field condenser instead of normal condenser which contains an opaque disc. The disc blocks those lights which enter the objective lens directly. Only the light that is reflected off (turned away from) the specimen enters the objective lens. The specimen appears bright against a dark background because there is no direct background light.

Construction and working

Various types of equipment's are used to produce dark field illumination that stop the light rays to pass through the specimen (Fig. 2.4), e.g. spider stop, placed underneath of condenser lens. This can also be accomplished by equipping light microscope with a special kind of condenser that transmits a hollow cone of light from the source of illumination, e.g. Abbe's dark field's condenser. There are two types of condenser:

1. Paraboloid condenser
2. Cardioid condenser

A dark field stop is kept in the condenser to prevent the entry of direct light. But when the light passes through the transparent specimen like microbial cells, it will be diffracted or scattered and this diffracted light will enter into the objective and reach the eye. Therefore the object or microbial cell will appear bright in a dark microscopic field.

Application

1. This technique is frequently used to examine the unstained microorganisms suspended in the liquid.

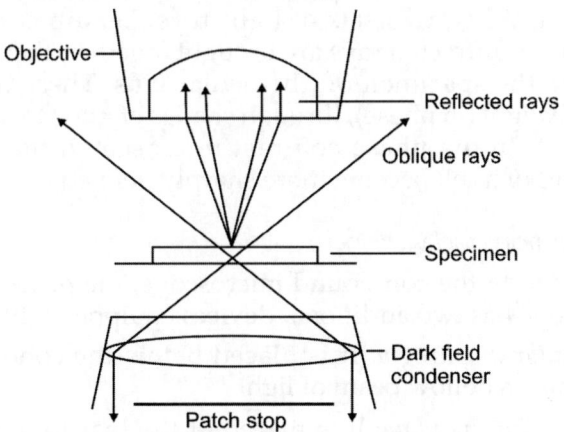

Fig. 2.4: Dark field microscope

2. Dark field microscopy is also used for the examination of very thin spirochetes, such as *Treponema pallidum*, the causative agent of syphilis.

3. Phase Contrast Microscope

The phase contrast microscopy is very useful because it permits the detailed examination of internal structure of living microorganisms. With this microscope, it is not necessary to fix or stain the specimen.

Principle

The microscopy is based on the wave nature of the light rays. It is based on the fact that light rays can be in phase (their peaks and valleys match) or out of phase. If the wave peak of light rays from the one source coincides with the wave peak of light rays from another source, the rays interact to produce reinforcement (relative brightness). If the wave peak from one light source coincides with the wave trough from another light source, the rays interact to produce interference (relative darkness). In a phase contrast microscope, one set of light rays comes directly from the light source. The other set comes from light that is reflected of diffracted from a particular structure in the specimen. Diffraction is the scattering of light rays as they touch a specimen's edge. The diffracted rays are bent away from the parallel light rays that pass farther from the specimen. When two sets of light rays, i.e. direct rays and refracted or diffracted rays are brought together, they form an image of the specimen on the ocular lens. These areas are relatively light (in phase), through shades of gray, to black (out of phase). In the phase contrast microscopy, the internal structures of a cell become more sharply defined.

Construction and working

In addition to the compound microscope, the phase contrast microscope has two additional devices equipped with it.

1. *Annular diaphragm:* It is placed below the condenser. It permits a hollow beam of light.

2. *Phase shifting plate:* It is placed at the rear focal plane of objective lens.

It is a disc composed of glass having circular coated area on it and is responsible for creating phase difference of ¼ wavelengths as compared to the light rays passing through the rest of the plate (Fig. 2.5).

Phase contrast light pathways

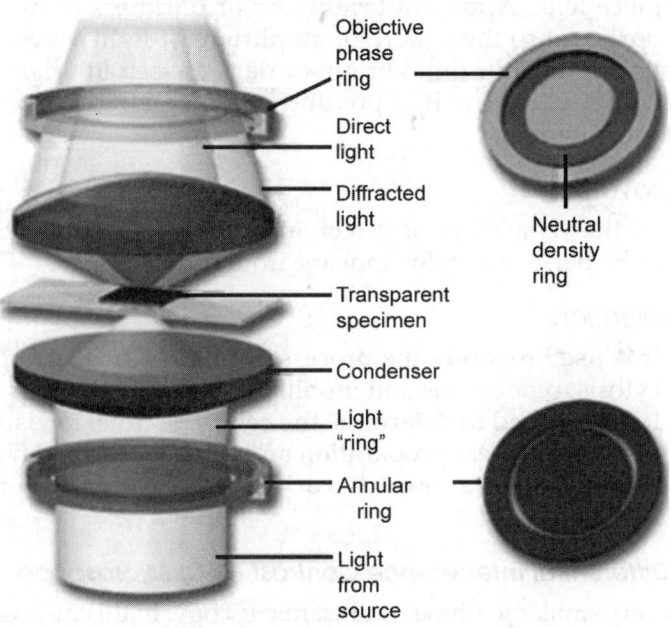

Fig. 2.5: Phase contrast microscopy

The source of light in the phase contrast microscope is visible light. Mirror reflects light towards the condenser. The condenser is equipped by special diaphragm, i.e. annular diaphragm. It allows only hollow beam of light. A hollow beam of light then strikes on the object. Depending on the internal details and refractive index of various components of object, certain rays get bended and are referred as diffracted rays (indirect rays), while certain rays travel in the straight line without any bending, called undiffracted rays (direct rays). Both the types of rays pass thorough objective and strike on the phase shifting plate. Here, undiffracted rays (direct rays) are passed through the phase ring (MgF coated region), on phase shifting plate and retarded or advanced the rays by ¼ wavelengths. While diffracted rays (indirect rays) pass through transparent region of the phase plate unchanged because they miss the phase ring, but these are already retarded by ¼ wavelength due to object. Finally, the rays including undiffracted rays and diffracted rays are brought together by eyepiece lens. Apparent brightness or darkness in image is proportional to the square of amplitude of light waves. The image will be four times bright or dark as seen in bright field microscope. Hence, it is possible to visualize the microbes without staining.

Disadvantage

Since, the separation of direct and diffracted light rays can never be perfect; a 'halo' appears around the object.

Application

1. It is used to study the process of mitosis, meiosis phago-cytosis, pinocytosis and motility of bacteria.
2. It is also used to determine the cell cycle time, to visualize unstained smear preparation and to study the behavior of living protozoa towards various physical and chemical factors.

4. Differential Interference Contrast (DIC) Microscope

It is very similar to phase contrast microscopy. In this microscopy, there are different refractive indexes that produce images.

Principle

DIC microscope uses two beam of light, separated by prisms. When contrasting colors are added by the prisms to the specimen, the specimen appears colored as a result of the prism effect. There is no staining required. The resolution of a DIC microscope is higher than that of a standard phase contrast microscope. Also, the image is brightly colored and appears nearly three dimensional.

Construction and working

This microscopy produces high contrast image of unstained transparent specimen in three-dimensional diagrams (Fig. 2.6).

The three special features are:
1. Polarizing filter
2. Interference contrast or Nomarski prism
3. Prism analyzer

In Nomarski differential interference microscopy, when polarized light pass through the prism, it splits into two beams that travels closely parallel to each other through the specimen (Fig. 2.6). When the light waves pass through the

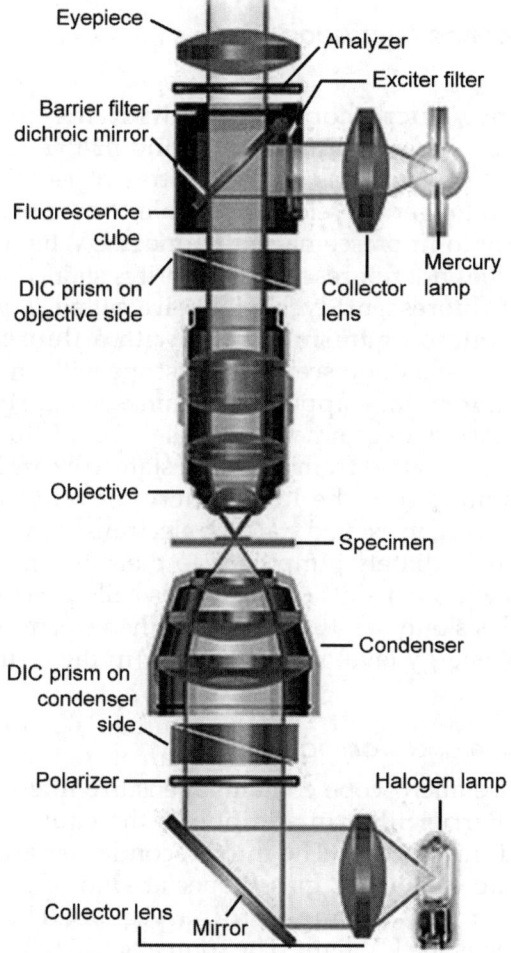

Fig. 2.6: Differential interference contrast (DIC) microscopy

specimen, their wave paths are altered due to varying thickness, slopes, refractive index. Now, when this light waves pass through auxiliary prism, they are recombined to produce interference pattern. Two combined beams of light are then allowed to pass through analyzer. As a result, a three-dimensional image is obtained, which is a function of refractive index differences at the boundary surface of the specimen. More will be the refractive index difference, larger will be the contrast.

5. Fluorescence Microscope

Principle

Fluorescence microscopy works with the principle of fluorescence. *Fluorescence* is the ability of the substance to absorb short wavelengths of light (Ultraviolet—UV) and give off light at a longer wavelength (visible). Some organism has the property to fluoresce naturally under UV light, but if the specimen does not fluoresce naturally, it is stained with one of a group of fluorescent dyes which are called *fluorochromes*. When the microorganism stained with a fluorochrome is examined under a fluorescence microscope with an UV or near UV light source, they appear as luminescent, bright objects against a dark background. The molecules of fluorochrome compound get excited from a ground state to excited state. The electron jumps from the lower energy level to the higher energy level. But in excited state the electrons are very unstable and they immediately jump back to their original state. (i.e. ground state). Such shift of electron is called 'Stroke's shift'. This state lasts only for 10^{-5} seconds. When electron returns to its original energy level it emits energy in the form of visible light.

Construction and working

Fluorescence microscope contains specialize filters: Excitation filter and Barrier filter in addition to the equipped parts of compound microscope. The mirror, condenser and objective are made up of 'Quartz glass' (special kind of glass), as UV light cannot pass through ordinary glass. The source of illumination is the UV light. The source of UV light is mercury arc or Xenon arc lamp.

Primary excitation filter is equipped near mercury lamp. It allows only the UV light of specific wavelength. The UV light is then reflected by mirror towards condenser. Condenser makes cone of light, which further strikes on the specimen. The specimen is self fluorescing or stained with flurochrome dye.

The UV rays strike on the specimen and get converted to visible light due to the phenomenon of fluorescence. Those UV rays which do, not strike on the specimen remains as UV rays. From this point, there are two types of rays which emerge out. As UV light is harmful for eye, the entry of these rays is restricted by specialized filter called as barrier filters (also called as secondary filter). These filters selectively allow visible light to pass through it and not UV light. Visible light further travels through eyepiece and is involved in image formation (Fig. 2.7).

Application

1. It is used to study the banding pattern of chromosomes and identification of chromosome, e.g. human Y-chromosome.
2. It is used in supravital staining: Staining the cells without killing the organism (living condition), is called supravital staining. The cells stained with such type of dyes can be easily detected with fluorescence microscope.
3. It is used to study the biological material like DNA, RNA, protein, carbohydrates, chlorophyll, etc.
4. Fluorescence antibody technique: Antigen or bacterial cells can be detected by flurochrome labeled antibody. This technique is known as Fluorescence Antibody (FA) technique.

6. Confocal Microscope

It is the recent development in the light microscopy. Like fluorescent microscopy, the specimen will be stained with fluorochromes and thus emits or return the light.

Principle

In this microscopy, one plane of a region of specimen is illuminated with a laser and passes the returned light through an aperture aligned with the illuminated region. Each plane corresponds to an image of fine slice that has been cut from

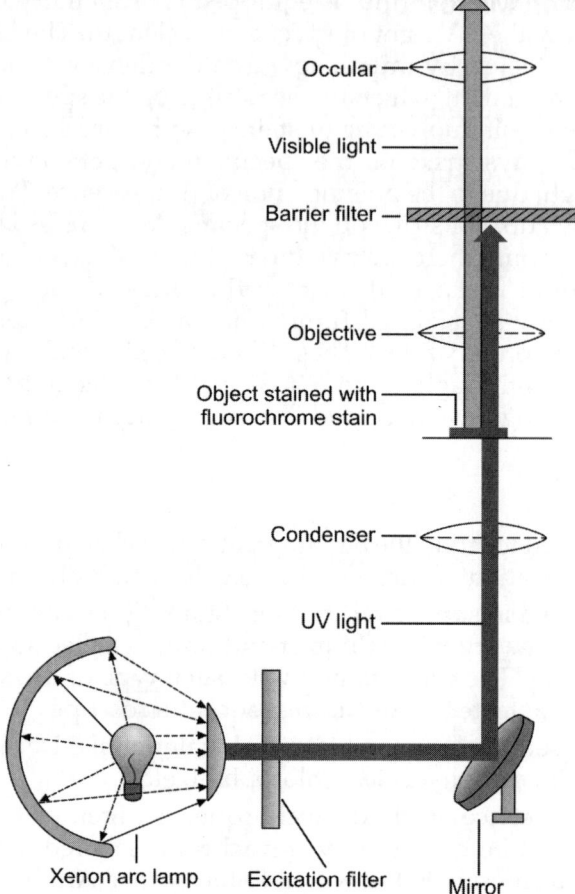

Fig. 2.7: The fluorescence microscope

specimen planes and regions are illuminated successively until the entire specimen has been scanned. Blurring is not the problem with this microscopy because confocal microscopy uses a pinhole aperture. As a resent, exponentially clear two dimensional images can be obtained and resolution of up to 40 % over that of the other microscope can be obtained. Most Confocal microscopes are used in conjunction with computers to obtain three-dimensional images of entire cells and cellular components. In addition, confocal microscopy is used to evaluate the cellular physiology.

B. Electron Microscopy

Knoll and *Ernest Ruska* (1931) developed the first electron microscope. It is used for the examination of the objects which are smaller than about 0.2 μm, such as viruses or the internal structures of the cells.

In the electron microscope, the beam of electrons is used as a source of illumination instead of light. Free electrons travel in the waves. The resolving power of the electron microscope is far greater than that of the other microscopes, it is due to the shorter wavelength of electrons; the wavelength of electrons are about 1,00,000 times smaller than the wavelengths of visible lights. Thus electron microscope is used to examine the structures which are too small to be resolved with the light microscope. Images produced by the electron microscopes are always black and white. Electron microscope uses the electromagnetic lenses instead of glass lenses to focus a beam of electrons onto a specimen. And the other functions are similar to that of the regular (optical) microscopes.

Application

1. *Topography*: To study the surface features of a sample
2. *Morphology*: To study the shape and size of particles making up the sample (cell organelles)
3. *Composition*: To identify the elements and compounds of the sample from which it is composed of and their amounts
4. *Crystallographic information*: How the atoms are arranged in the sample

Steps involved

A stream of electrons is formed and they are accelerated towards the sample with the help of positive electrical potential. The stream of electrons is focused using metallic apertures and magnetic lenses to produce a thin and focused monochromatic beam. The interaction with the sample affects the beam, which is then detected and transformed into the image.

Types of electron microscopy

1. Transmission Electron Microscope
2. Scanning Electron Microscope

1. Transmission Electron Microscope

Principle

The source of illumination in this microscopy is the electron beam. The resolution of the microscope depends on the wavelength of light. Hence, using the low wavelength is responsible for increasing resolution. Electron beam used in this microscope has wavelength of 5 nm as compared to wavelength of light rays, i.e. 280 to 800 nm. If the system gives the highest resolution, the magnification can also be increased by 10^5. The transmission electron microscope is so called because the electron beam travels through the thin specimen. The rest of principle is relatively similar to that of the light microscope.

Construction

The transmission electron microscope consists of following parts:

1. *Electron gun:* The source of illumination in this microscope is electron beam which is generated by the electron gun; it is located at the top of the microscope. The high voltage electricity is supplied to the tungsten filament to form electron beam. This tungsten filament is surrounded by cathode plate which consists of aperture, through which the electron beam is drawn towards anode.

2. *Microscope column:* It consists of an evacuated metal tube. The series of electromagnetic lenses, viewing screen and photographic plate are placed one above the other. The microscope column provides a protective shield to the operator from X-rays and other harmful radiation that are generated when the electron strikes the metal surface.

3. *Vacuum pump:* The microscopic column is maintained under vacuum. If the vacuum is not applied, the electron beam gets scattered easily by the dust particles and molecules of air. Cooling system is also equipped to compensate high heat generated by the system.

4. *Electromagnetic lenses:* Electron microscope uses electromagnetic lenses as a lens system. Each coil has electric wire wound on a hollow metal cylinder to form an axially symmetrical magnetic field. The electron beam passes

through the microscope column and gets deflected by the various degrees depending on the current flowing in coil of lens. The magnetic field functions as 'magnetic lenses.

5. *Fluorescent screen:* The magnified image is viewed in the form of fluorescence screen because the direct electrons are harmful for observer's eyes. The image can also be observed on photographic plate placed below the projector lens.

Preparation of specimen for TEM

Biological specimen containing water cannot simply be placed in high vacuum because the water will boil off, destroying the integrity of organism. Therefore before viewing it must be dehydrated to fix the structure by placing in acetone or alcohol. The specimen is then placed in dilute solution of plastic embedding material and the plastic is polymerized. The sections of hard plastic block containing specimen is cut be ultra-microtome. Sections are collected, stained and placed on a copper grid to view in electron microscope.

Working

The electrons are used for magnification and image formation and also for better resolution because the electrons have a much shorter wavelength. The source of illumination is electron beam which is generated by electron gun. The electrons in the form of beams are passed through the condenser coil. They get scattered and transmitted through the objects and pass through the objective coil; these magnifies the image of the object (Fig. 2.8).

The projector coil further magnifies the image and projects it on the fluorescent screen or photographic film. When the energy of electrons is transformed into visible light through the excitation of chemical coating of the screen, the image formation occurs. These electrons, which reach the fluorescent screen, form the bright spots while the areas where electrons do not reach the screen form the dark spots.

The area which scattered electron is termed as 'electron dense'. Electron strikes the atomic nuclei and gets dispersed and forms the image. The electron image thus formed is converted into visible form by projecting on the fluorescence

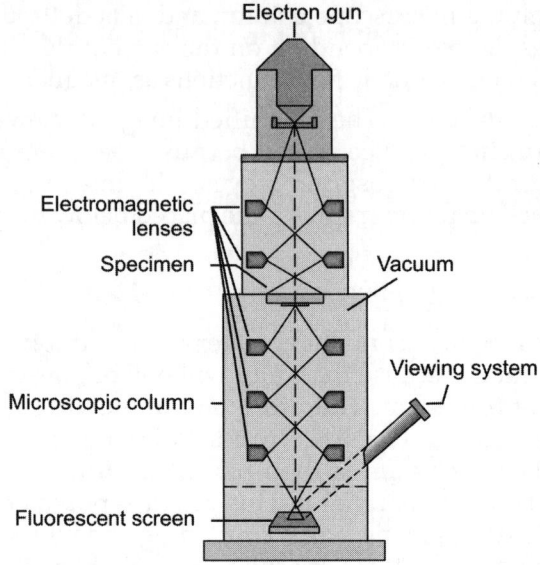

Fig. 2.8: The transmission electron microscope

screen. Electron dispersion is due to atomic nuclei, which consist of protons and neutrons. The higher the atomic number greater will be the dispersion. Since the biological material generally have low atomic number, the dispersion of electrons is poor which causes poor contrast in image. Thus, to improve the contrast in the image salts of heavy metals are used for staining the specimen.

Magnification

Electron microscope fitted with intermediate coil can get a magnification up to 1,60,000X. This magnification can be further increased by microphotography up to 10 lakhs times without the loss of sharpness.

Resolving power

The resolution of electron microscope is 0.4–1 nm.

2. Scanning Electron Microscope

The scanning electron microscope was built by *Van Ardene* (1938) who inserted scanning coil in the microscope.

Principle

Here, the electron beam is not transmitted through specimen but impinges on its surface from above; by this way it differs from the transmission electron microscope. A narrow beam of electrons with the high velocity from an electron gun passes through condenser lenses and other magnetic lenses. This produce and focus an electron beam or probe of 5–10 nm diameter as a spot on the specimen surface. The electron probe, which scans over the specimen surface, excites the specimen molecule to emit the energy. This energy is released by excited molecule in several form including high energy electrons which are called 'secondary electrons'.

The number of secondary electrons released depends on angle of specimen point on which the electron beam or probe is reflected. These secondary electrons are deflected towards collector and deflector. The successive electric signals are amplified and transmitted to cathode tube. The scanning beam and cathode ray beam are synchronized and the image can be observed on the TV screen (Fig. 2.9).

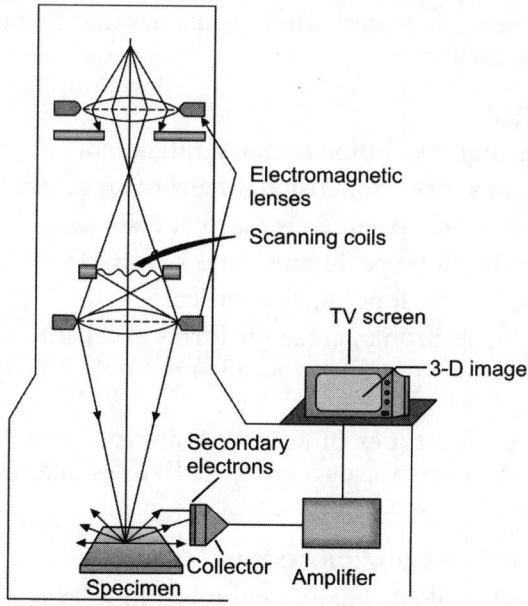

Fig. 2.9: The scanning electron microscope

Construction and working

The electron beam comes from the hot tungsten or Lanthanum hexaboride cathode gun. The electron beam is too broad so it is to be narrowed and adjusted by magnetic lens. The sharp probe of about 5–10 nm diameter is made from the electron beam. This probe covers the 5–10 nm area on specimen at a time.

The electron probe enters to the great depth and then moved rapidly back and front in simple harmonic motion or scan over the specimen surface by scanning coil and beam deflector. This attracts the electron beam of magnetic system. The electron probe that scans the specimen surface at each time excites the molecule to high energy level. This energy is released in the form of 'secondary electrons'. The secondary electron with sufficient energy is deflected toward deflector placed towards one side of the specimen and converts them into pulses of electric current.

In some systems, scintillation counter is placed to convert the energy of secondary electron to electric current. The current with low pulses are amplified by amplifier and finally pass through the cathode ray tube. The scanning electron beam is synchronized with cathode ray tube so that 3-D image can be continuously seen.

Advantages

- It gives high resolution and magnification.
- It provides three-dimensional view of an object.
- Preparation of specimen is rapid and simple.
- Relatively short specimen time is required.
- It is used in the topological studies.
- Scanning electron microscope forms excellent image of the object surface ranging in size from whole cell up to small insect.

Recently, two types of scanning microscopes have been discovered. The microscopy is called as scanned probe microscopy.

C. Scanned Probe Microscopy

Since period of 1980s, many new types of microscopes called scanned probe microscopes have been developed.

They use various types of probes for the examination of surface of specimen at very close range. It is done without modifying the specimen. These types of microscopes can be used to observe atomic and molecular shapes to characterize magnetic and chemical properties and to determine temperature variation inside the cells. They are classified into two groups:

1. Scanning tunneling microscopy
2. Atomic force microscopy

1. Scanning Tunneling Microscopy (STM)

Here, the thin metal (tungsten) probe scans the specimen and produces an image that reveals the bumps and depressions on the surface of the specimen. The resolving power of STM is much greater than that of the electron microscope. It can resolve the features of about 1/100 the size of an atom. Moreover, for observation, special preparation of specimen is not required. STMs are used to view and observe the molecules such as DNA.

2. Atomic Force Microscopy (AFM)

Here, the metal and diamond probe is gently forced down onto a specimen. As the probe moves along the surface of specimen, its movements are recorded and three dimensional images are formed. Like STM; AFM also does not require special preparation for specimen. AFM is used to image both, the biological (in nearly atomic detail) and molecular forces (such as assembly of fibrin, a component of blood clot).

II. STAINING TECHNIQUE

A. Definition

Stain is defined as an organic compound containing both the chromophore and auxochrome groups, while color contains only the chromphoric group. Practically, staining the bacteria enhances the contrast. Stains are natural or artificial organic compounds. Chromophore group imparts colour to stain. Any substance, which possesses only chromophore group, is not a stain. But it must have affinity to bind with cells or tissues. The group that imparts ability to bind cells or tissues is called auxochrome. The electrolytic dissociation of auxochrome group helps to bind the stain to cell, e.g. nitrobenzene is a color while picric acid is a dye (NO_2 is chromophore while phenolic group is auxochrome).

B. Importance of Staining

1. Microbes are semitransparent because the refractive index of microbes is approximately equal to the refractive index of the surrounding environment. So, to increase the visibility and to develop the better contrast with surrounding, staining is an essential step.
2. It is important for studying the morphology (shape and size) of microbe.
3. It is also helpful in detecting the extracellular and intracellular components of microbe. (Capsule, spore and flagella, etc.)
4. Staining is also clinically important. It is helpful for primary level of identification. (If the bacteria is gram-positive/gram-negative or acid-fast/non-acid-fasts) which is also important in diagnosis and to determine the course of treatment.

C. Theories of Staining

The staining can be explained on the basis of combination of both the given theories, i.e. physical and chemical

a. **Physical theory:** It suggests that all the staining reactions can be explained on the basis of various physical reactions like osmosis, adsorption and absorption. A physical process is a reaction between two substances without the formation of new compound. When the bacteria are stained, the stain will not be changed chemically to form a new compound. It is possible to extract the stain from cells by water or alcohol.

b. **Chemical theory:** The chemical theory suggests that staining is a chemical reaction that occurs between bacterial cell component and stain molecule. The bacterial cell possesses the slightly negative charge. The cationic stain is with basic—chromophore groups, on dissociation the stain forms positive ion. Such positive ion binds to bacterial cell, which possesses a negative charge.

D. Classification of Stains

Depending upon the positive or negative electrical charge present on chromophore, stains are grouped as acidic stains and basic stains.

a. **Acidic stain (anionic stain):** A stain, which possesses the negatively charged chromophore, is acidic stain or stain on ionization gives negatively charged molecule. The chromophore has negative charge. It is repelled by negatively charged cell. It tends to stain area of slide around the cell, e.g. sodium eosinate, nigrosine, Congo red, rose Bengal stain, etc.

b. **Basic stain (cationic stain):** The stain that possesses the positively charged chromophore is basic stain or a stain which are on ionization gives positively charged molecule. The chromophore has positive charge that attracted towards negatively charged cell. It tends to stain cell, e.g. methylene blue, crystal violet, safranin, malachite green, etc.

c. **Leuco compound:** It is the stains which on reduction of chromophore group forms loss of colour are called leuco compound.

d. **Mordant:** A mordant may be defines as any substance that forms an insoluble compound with stain and serves to fix the colour to bacterial cell, e.g. acid mordant—alum, ferrous sulphate, etc. Basic mordant—picric acid, tannic acid, etc.

E. Types of Staining

1. Simple Staining

a. Negative/indirect (relief) staining

Principle: The bacterial morphology can be studied by negative staining. Negative staining is also referred as indirect or relief staining. Negative staining is the technique in which background is stained and the cell remains colourless.

The bacterial cell possesses slight negative charge. The acidic stain is used in this staining (e.g. eosin stain, nigrosine, Congo red, rose Bengal stain, etc. Such stain is not responsible for the staining of the cell because there is repulsion between two similar charges, i.e. negative charge of acidic stain and negatively charged bacterial cell. But it will bind with the positively charged glass slide. Some other stains having molecular size greater than bacterial pores are also useful in such staining (e.g. India ink). The stain particle remains outside the cell and just stains the background.

Procedure

- Wash the glass slide with detergent and water to remove all the dirt and grease. Handle this cleaned slide by its edges throughout the performance of an experiment.
- Take a loopful amount of bacterial suspension at the right edge of the clean slide with the help of an inoculating loop.
- Add the drop of nigrosine solution to the bacterial suspension and mix it. Do not spread the drop during this mixing.
- Spread the mixture using a second slide (spreader slide), while spreading hold the slide at an angle of 45°C, so that a thin film of bacterial suspension is formed.
- Allow to dry the film.
- Observe the slide under oil immersion objective.

Advantages

1. The negative staining is generally used for bacteria which are difficult to stain, e.g. *Spirilla*.
2. This technique does not distort the morphology of bacteria as there are no harsh physical (e.g. heating) or chemical treatments.

b. Monochrome staining

Principle: Single stain to colour the bacteria is commonly referred to as monochrome staining. (Mono means single and chrome means colour.) While using this method it is to be kept in the mind that the bacteria possess slight negative charge. The negatively charged group of bacterial cell surface produces attraction between the basic stains. Stains used commonly in this method are methylene blue, crystal violet, etc.

Procedure

- Wash the glass slide with the detergent and water to remove all the dirt and grease. Handle this cleaned slide by it sedges throughout the performance of practical.
- Draw a half-inch (approx. 1.5 cm) circle on the centre of the slide. Then invert the slide.
- Take a loop-full of bacterial suspension on the centre of slide and then spread throughout the circle uniformly.

- Allow the slide to air dry by normal evaporation of water.
- After the drying of smear pass the slide through Bunsen burner flame, to heat fix the microorganisms to the slide.
- Stain the bacterial suspension with appropriate stain. Staining should be done in the staining rack near the sink or preferably in a koplin jar. The slide should be covered with the stain for appropriate time period.
- Briefly wash the stain from the slide with gentle flow of tap water.
- Allow the slide to air dry.
- Observe the slide under oil immersion objective.

2. Differential Staining Technique

The staining technique, which differentiates two kinds of microbes, is known as differential staining technique. The stains used in this method react differently with various microbes. The differentiation is due to the chemical composition of organisms. Differentiation staining techniques involves gram stain and Acid-fast stain. The differential staining is generally used to determine morphology, e.g. cell wall, cell membrane, capsules, endotoxins, or exotoxins and hence allows detailed characterization of bacteria.

a. Gram staining

Principle: The cell wall of gram-positive bacteria contains magnesium ribonucleate and negligible amount of lipids. The cell wall of gram-negative bacteria contains high percentage of lipids and it lacks magnesium ribonucleate. The primary stain crystal violet is responsible for staining both the kinds of cells.

In second step, a mordant, i.e. gram's iodine is added. It leads to form crystal violet-iodine-magnesium ribonucleate complex in gram-positive bacteria. This complex is not formed in gram-negative bacteria because the magnesium-ribonucleate is absent in their cell wall.

In the next step, the decolourizer (70% alcohol) is responsible for the extraction of lipids from the gram-negative bacteria. The lipid is a major component of these cells. Removal of lipid makes the cell porous, which further allows release of crystal violet from cytoplasm.

Gram-negative cell become colourless at this step. In case of gram-positive bacteria, lipids are absent and above consequence will never occur. Thus, the gram-positive cell still retains crystal violet and appears as violet. The counter stain safranin is responsible to stain gram-negative bacteria. As safranin is basic stain it also partially stains the gram-positive cell to negligible extent and imparts purple color. Hence, under oil immersion objective we can observe purple-coloured gram-positive bacteria and pink-colored gram-negative bacteria.

Procedure

- Prepare a smear from the bacterial suspension on a clean grease free slide, fix it with heat.
- Cover the smear by crystal violet and keep for 1 minute
- Wash the stain with distilled water by using a wash bottle
- Cover the smear with grams iodine and keep it for 1 minute
- Pour off the grams iodine and flood the smear with 70% alcohol till the solvent flows in colourless solution.
- This step is important because thick smears require more time than thin ones. Decolourization occurs when solvent flows colourlessly.
- Stop the action of alcohol by rinsing the slide with water.
- Cover the smear with basic stain safranin for 1 minute and then wash the slide under gentle flow of water and allow the slide to air dry.
- Observe the slide under oil immersion objective.

b. Acid-fast staining

Many bacteria do not get decolorized even after the application of a strong decolorizer like acid-alcohol mixture; this property is known as acid-fastness. Acid-fast staining technique is a differential staining technique that categorizes the bacteria into acid-fast and non-acid-fast.

This staining is useful in the diagnosis of tuberculosis bacilli *Mycobacterium tuberculosis* which is an acid-fast bacteria.

Principle: Several kinds of bacteria like *Mycobacterium* species and many *Actinomycetes* contain mycolic acid and other waxy material in their cell wall. Such bacteria do not get stained with ordinary staining techniques.

The chemical composition makes the cell impermeable to stains. If such a cell is stained with potent stain like Ziehl Neelsen carbol-fuchsin along with steaming, it gets stained. The acid fast microorganisms retain the red colour because the carbol-fuchsin is more soluble in the cell wall lipids than in the acid-alcohol. In the next step, when a strong decolourized acid-alcohol is added to such a stained smear, non-acid-fast bacteria, whose cell walls lack the lipid components, the carbol-fuchsin is rapidly removed during decolourinzation, leaving the cell colorless. The use of counter stain methylene blue is responsible to stain these colourless cells. Finally the acid-fast bacteria appear pink and non-acid-fast bacteria appear blue.

Procedure

- Prepare a smear of given bacterial suspension on a clean, dried glass slide.
- Flood the smear with carbol-fuchsin stain. At the same time, hold the slide on boiling water bath for five minutes. Add the stain if slide become dry.
- After five minutes, allow the slide to cool.
- Add decolourizer acid-alcohol mixture for three seconds. Stop the action of decolourizer by rinsing the slide with tap water.
- Add the counter stain methylene blue for one minute.
- Wash the slide with tap water. Allow the slide to air dry. Observe the slide under oil immersion objective.

3. Special Staining

Special stains are used to colour and isolate the specific parts of microorganisms, such as endospores and flagella and to reveal the presence of capsules.

a. Negative staining for capsules

Many microorganisms contain a gelatinous covering called a capsule. Capsule staining is more difficult than other types of staining procedures because capsular materials are soluble in water and may be removed during rigorous washing.

To observe the presence of capsules, a microbiologist can mix the bacteria in a solution containing a fine colloidal suspension of colored particles (commonly, India ink or nigrosin) to provide a dark background and then stain the bacteria with a simple stain, such as safranin (Fig. 2.10).

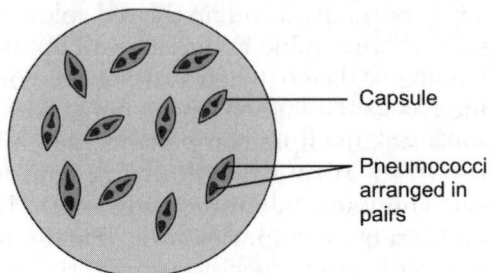

Fig. 2.10: Capsule staining

Because of their chemical composition, capsules do not accept most biological dyes, such as safranin and thus appear as halos surrounding, stained with bacterial cell.

b. Endospore (spore) staining

An endospore is a special resistant, dormant structure formed within a cell that protects a bacterium from adverse environmental conditions. Endospores cannot be stained by ordinary methods, such as simple staining and gram staining, because the dyes do not penetrate the wall of the endospore. The most commonly used endospore stain is the Schaeffer-Fulton endospore stain.

Procedure

- Malachite green, the primary stain is applied to a heat fixed smear and heated to steaming for about 5 minutes. The heat helps the stain to penetrate the endospore wall.
- Then the preparation is washed for about 30 seconds with water to remove the malachite green from all of the cells parts except the endospores.
- Next, safranin, a counter stain, is applied to the smear to stain portions of the cell other than endospores.

Observation

In a properly prepared smear, the endospores appear green within red or pink cells. Because endospores are highly refractive, they can be detected under the light microscope when unstained, but they cannot be differentiated from inclusions of stored material without a special stain.

c. Flagella staining

Bacterial flagella are the structures which are too small to be seen with the light microscope without staining. A tedious and delicate staining procedure uses a mordant and the stain carbol-fuchsin to build up the diameter of flagella until they become visible under the light microscope. Microbiologists use the number and arrangement of flagella as diagnostic aids.

III. CLASSIFICATION OF TAXONOMY

It is the science of classifying organisms that permits logical and informative system of naming and is useful for the identification of an organism.

Classification: It is the assignment of organisms into an organized scheme of naming.

A. Major Characteristics Used in Classification

1. Morphological characters
2. Physiological and metabolic characters
3. Ecological characters
4. Molecular or genetic characters

B. General Methods Used in Classification of Microorganism

1. Intuitive Method

A microbiologist who is thoroughly familiar with the properties of the group of microorganism may decide to pool those organisms into one species or genera. The disadvantage with this method is that the characteristics he used for classification may be important to him and may not be so important to another.

2. Numerical Taxonomy

In this method many characteristics for each strain studied. Then percentage of similarity of each strain to every other strain is calculated. According to the percentage of similarity, microorganisms are grouped into species.

C. Prokaryotic and Eukaryotic Cells

Distinguishing features between Prokaryotic cells and Eukaryotic cells are given below:

Feature	Prokaryotic cells	Eukaryotic cells
Groups where found as unit of structure	Bacteria	Algae, fungi, protozoa, plants, and animals
Size range of organism	1 – 2 by 1– 4 µm or less	Greater than 5 µm in width or diameter
General characteristics of bacteria		
Genetic system		
Location	Nucleoid, chromatin body, or nuclear material	Nucleus, mitochondria, chloroplasts
Structure of nucleus	Not bounded by nuclear membrane; one circular chromosome	Bounded by nuclear membrane; more than one chromosome
	Chromosome does not contain histones; no mitotic division	Chromosomes have histones; mitotic nuclear division
	Nucleolus absent; functionally related genes may be clustered	Nucleolus present; functionally related genes not clustered
Sexuality	Zygote nature is merozygotic (partial diploid)	Zygote is diploid
Cytoplasmic nature and structures		
Cytoplasmic	Absent	Present streaming
Pinocytosis	Absent	Present
Gas vacuoles	Can be present	Absent
Mesosome	Present	Absent
Ribosomes	70S distributed in the cytoplasm	80S arrayed on membranes as in endoplasmic reticulum; 70S in mitochondria and chloroplasts

(Contd...)

(Contd...)

Feature	Prokaryotic cells	Eukaryotic cells
Mitochondria	Absent	Present
Chloroplasts	Absent	May be present
Golgi structures	Absent	Present
Endoplasmic reticulum	Absent	Present
Membrane-bound (true) vacuoles	Absent	Present
Outer cell structures		
Cytoplasmic membranes	Generally do not contain sterols; contain part of respiratory and, in some, photosynthetic machinery	Sterols present; do not carry out respiration and photosynthesis
Cell wall	Peptidoglycan (murein or mucopeptide) as component	Absence of peptidoglycan
Locomotor organelles	Simple fibril	Multifibrilled with 9 + 2 microtubules

IV. BACTERIA

A. General Characteristics of Bacteria

Bacteria are unicellular, free-living, microscopic microorganisms capable of performing all the essential functions of life. They possess both deoxyribonucleic acid (DNA) and ribonucleic acid (RNA). Bacteria are prokaryotic micro-organisms that do not contain chlorophyll. They occur in water, soil, air, food and all natural environments. They can survive extremes of temperature, pH, oxygen tension and atmospheric pressures. They are very small which are visible under the light microscope. Generally, *Cocci* are about 1 μm in diameter and bacilli are 1 to 8 μm in length and 0.1 to 0.5 μm in width.

B. Classification of Bacteria

Bacteria are classified as follows:

i. Based on shape (Fig. 2.11)

On the basis of shape, bacteria are classified as follows:

1. **Cocci:** They are small, spherical or oval cells. In Greek, *'kokkos'* means 'berry'.

2. **Bacilli:** They are derived from the Greek word *'Bacillum'* meaning 'stick'. They are rod-shaped cells, e.g. *Bacillus anthracis*.

    Coccobacilli: in some of the bacilli the length of the cells may be equal to the width. Such bacillary forms are known as Coccobacilli, e.g. *Bracella*.

3. **Vibrios:** They are comma-shaped, curved rods, e.g. *Vibrio comma*.

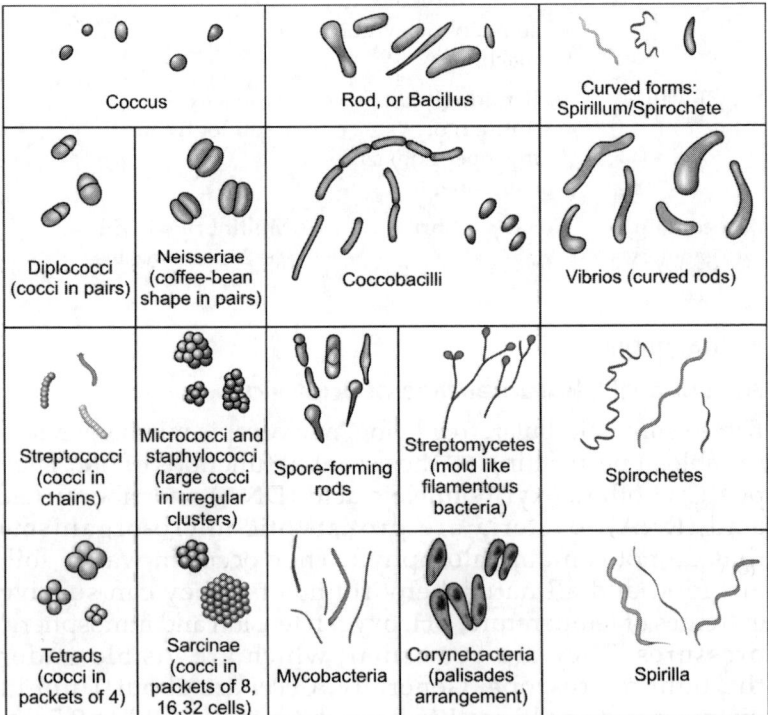

Fig. 2.11: Classification of bacteria according to their shapes

4. **Spirilla:** They are longer rigid rods with several curves or coils. They have a helical shape and rapid bodies, e.g. *Spirillum rubrum.*

5. **Spirochetes:** They are slender and flexuous spiral forms.

6. **Actinomycetes:** They are branching filamentous bacteria. The characteristic shape is due to the presence of a rigid cell wall, e.g. *Streptomyces* species.

7. **Mycoplasmas:** They are cell wall deficient bacteria and hence do not possess a stable morphology. They occur as round or oval bodies with interlacing filaments.

ii. Based on arrangement of bacterial cells (Fig. 2.12)

Cocci appear in several characteristic arrangement or groupings.

1. **Diplococci:** Cocci that split along one plane only, tend to arrange themselves in pair, e.g. *Diplococcus pneumoniae.*

2. **Streptococci:** These cells divide in one plane and remain attached, to form chains, e.g. *Lactococcus lactis.*

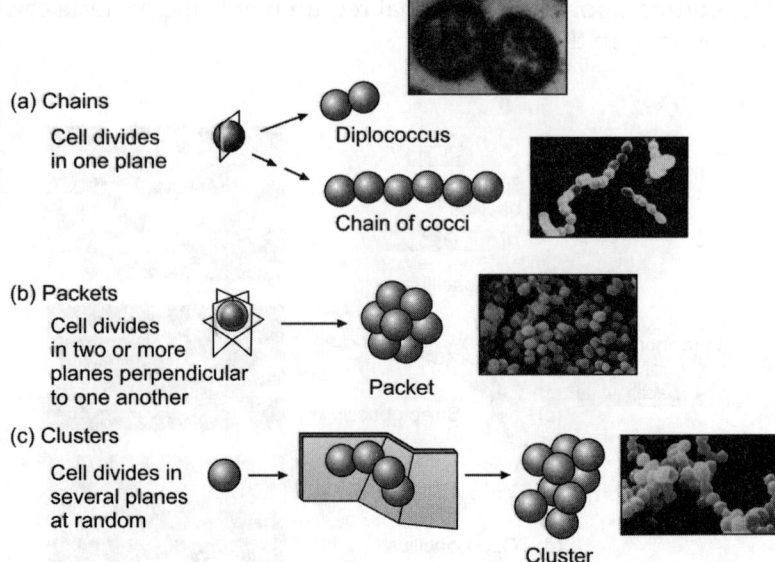

(a) Chains

Cell divides in one plane

Diplococcus

Chain of cocci

(b) Packets

Cell divides in two or more planes perpendicular to one another

Packet

(c) Clusters

Cell divides in several planes at random

Cluster

Fig. 2.12: Classification of bacteria according to arrangement of cells (cocci)

3. **Tetracocci:** They divide in two planes and live in groups of four, e.g. *Gaffkya tetragena*.

4. **Staphylococci:** Cocci cells divide in three planes in an irregular pattern. These cells produce bunches of cocci as in grapes, e.g. *Staphylococcus aureus*.

5. **Sarcinae:** They divide in three planes in a regular pattern. These cells produce a cuboidal arrangement of group of an eight cells.

Bacilli split only across their short axis. Arrangements of groupings formed by bacilli species are limited (Fig. 2.13).

1. **Diplobacilli:** They may appear as pairs, e.g. *Klebsiella pneumoniae*.

2. **Streptobacilli:** Some species are found in chains, e.g. *Bacillus subtilis*.

3. **Trichomes:** Some species forms trichomes, which are similar to chains but have a much large area of contact between the adjacent cells e.g. *Beggiatoa* and *Saprospira*.

iii. Based on nutritional requirements

Depending upon the nutritional requirements the bacteria can be classified in three groups:

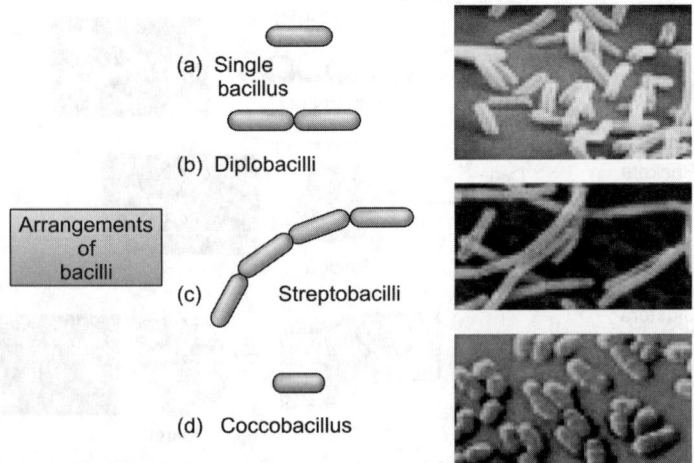

Fig. 2.13: Classification of bacteria according to their shapes (bacilli)

a. Based on source of energy

1. **Chemotrophs:** Some microbes rely on the chemical compounds for their energy and known as chemotrophs, e.g. *Escherichia coli.*

2. **Prototroph:** Some microbes utilize radiant energy (sunlight) and are called as phototrophs, e.g. *Rhodospirillum rubrum.*

b. Based on source of electron

All the microbes require electrons for their metabolism. They are classified as below.

1. **Lithotrophs:** Some organisms can use reduced inorganic compounds as electron donors and are termed as lithotrophs (some may be chemolithotrophs and others may be photolithotrophs), e.g. *Pseudomonas pseudoflava.*

2. **Organotrophs:** Some organism uses organic compound as an electron donor and are called organotrophs (some may be chemoorganotrophs and others photoorganotrophs), e.g. *Escherichia coli.*

c. Based on carbon requirement

All microorganisms require carbon for synthesizing cell components.

1. **Autotrophs:** some microorganism use carbon dioxide as their major or even sole, source of carbon and are termed as autotrophs, e.g. *Chromatium okenii.*

2. **Heterotrophs:** Some microbes require organic compound as their carbon source are termed as heterotrophs, e.g. *Escherichia coli.*

iv. Based on gaseous requirements

Bacteria display a wide variety of response to free oxygen. It is convenient to divide them into four groups on the following bases (Fig. 2.14):

1. **Aerobic bacteria:** They require oxygen for growth and can grow when they are incubated in an air atmosphere (i.e. 21% oxygen).

2. **Anaerobic bacteria:** They do not use oxygen to obtain energy; moreover, oxygen is toxic for them. They cannot grow when incubated in an air atmosphere.

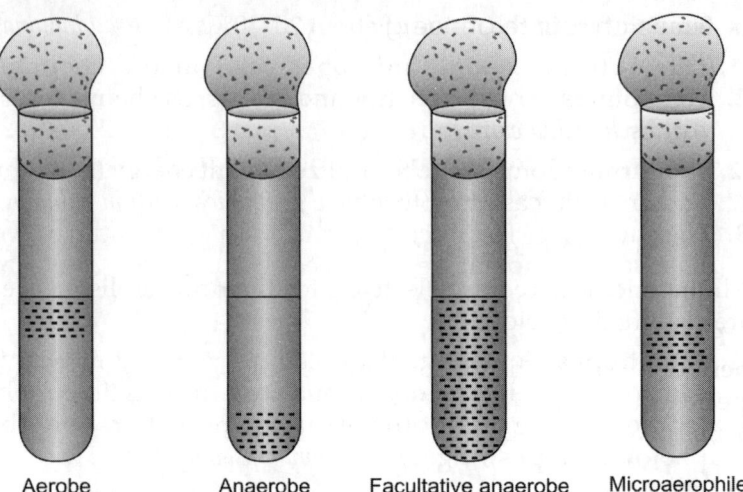

Aerobe   Anaerobe   Facultative anaerobe   Microaerophile

Fig. 2.14: Classification of bacteria according to Gaseous

Non-stringent/tolerant anaerobes: They are those that tolerate low levels of oxygen.

Stringent/strict anaerobes: They are those that cannot tolerate even low levels and may die upon brief exposure to air.

3. **Facultative anaerobic bacteria:** They do not require oxygen for growth; still they may use the oxygen for energy production if it is available. They are not inhibited by oxygen and usually grow well under an air atmosphere as like they grow in the absence of oxygen.

4. **Microaerophilic bacteria:** They require low levels of oxygen for growth but cannot tolerate the level of oxygen present in an air atmosphere.

v. Based on temperature requirement

On the basis of their temperature relationship, bacteria can be divided into three main groups.

1. **Psychrophiles:** The organism that can grow at 0°C but have a optimum temperature 15°C or lower and maximum temperature of 20°C. e.g. *Vibrio psychroerythrus.*

   Psychrotrophic (facultative psychrophile): Organism, that are able to grow at 0°C but which grow best at temperature in the range of about 20–30°C, e.g. *Pseudomonas fluorescens*.

2. **Mesophiles:** These are those organisms that grow best within a temperature range of approximately 25 –40°C. Most bacteria are growing best at about body temperature (37°C), e.g. *Corynebacterium diphtheriae*.

3. **Thermophiles:** The microbes which can grow and survive at elevated temperature are called thermophiles. They are those which grow best at temperature above 45°C.

Facultative thermophiles: The growth range of many thermophilic bacteria extends to the mesophilic region. These species are called as facultative thermophiles, e.g. *Streptococcus thermophilus*.

True/obligate/steno thermophiles: The thermophilic bacteria which requires essentially high temperatures for growth and cannot grow in mesophilic range are termed as true/obligate/steno thermophiles, e.g. *Thermus aquaticus*.

vi. Based on pH

Depending upon the optimum pH value of microorganisms, they can be classified as follows:

1. **Acidophiles:** These microorganisms have an optimum pH range in between 1 and 6.5, e.g. *Thiobacillus thiooxidans* (pH 2–3.5).

2. **Neutrophils:** Most bacteria grow best in a narrow pH range between 6.5 and 7.5. Such bacteria are called neutrophils, e.g. *Escherichia coli, Salmonella typhi*, all pathogenic bacteria.

3. **Alkaliphiles:** These microorganisms have an optimum pH range in between 7.5 and 14, e.g. *Vibrio cholerae* (pH 9).

V. ACTINOMYCETES

"Actino" meaning rays and "mycetes" means fungus. They are aerobic, gram-positive bacteria that form branching filaments or hyphae and asexual spores. Their morphology and arrangement of spores, cell wall chemistry and the types of sugar present in cell extracts are particularly important in actinomycete taxonomy. Actinomycetes have considerable impact on soil microbiology as they play important role in mineralization of organic matter in the soil.

A. General Characteristics of Actinomycetes

1. They have prokaryotic cell.
2. These are filamentous bacteria, morphologically they resemble to fungi. The filaments of actinomycetes are thinner than fungal filaments.
3. Several actinomycetes contain mycolic acid and waxy material in their cell wall along with peptidoglycan (acid-fast cell wall).
4. The genus *Frankia* has capacity to fix atmospheric nitrogen.
5. The members of Streptomyces produce gaseous compound geosmin, which gives typical fragrance of soil and can be experienced during first rain shower.
6. Reproduction of actinomycetes is by fragmentation, formation of asexual spores and by binary fission.
7. On the solid substrate, actinomycetes develop branching network of hyphae both on the surface and in the surface of substrate form substrate mycelium.
8. Septa usually divide the hyphae into long cells containing several nucleoids.
9. Sometimes they develop thallus (tissue like erect mass).
10. Aerial mycelium extends above the substratum and forms asexual, thin walled spores.
11. Most actinomycetes are not motile.

Significance

They are primarily soil inhabitants and are widely distributed. They can degrade on enormous number and variety of organic compounds. They produce most of the medically useful natural antibiotics, e.g. Streptomycin, Chloramphenicol, Neomycin, etc. Actinomycosis is a very chronic disease characterized by multiple abscesses, granuloma, tissue destruction, fibrosis and sinusitis.

Classification

Actinomycetes are classified as below:

1. Actinomycetaceae
2. Streptomycetaceae, e.g. *Streptomyces griseus*

3. Actinoplanaceae, e.g. *Actinoplanes*
4. Nocardiaceae, e.g. *Nocardia asteroides*
5. Micromonospora: Produce gentamicin
6. Dermatophilaceae, e.g. *Dermatophilus*

Streptomyces

Streptomyces have aerial hyphae divided in a single plane to form chains of 5 to 50 or more non mobile condiospores with surface texture ranging from smooth to spiny.

Ecological and medical importance

Streptomyces are known for the synthesis of vast variety of antibiotics which includes amphotericin B, chloramphenicol, erythromycin, streptomycin, tetracycline, etc. Streptomycetes play a major role in mineralization. They are flexible; nutritionally and aerobically degrade substrate like pectin, chitin, keratin, lignin, latex and aromatic compounds. The natural habitat of streptomycetes is soft where they may constitute from 1–20% of the culturable population.

B. Examples of Actinomycetes

Actinoplanes, Arthrobacter, Bifidobacterium, Corynebacterium, Frankia, Mycobacterium, Nocardia, Propionibacterium, Streptomyces.

VI. FUNGI

Fungi include eukaryotic spore-bearing organisms, no chlorophyll, reproduce both sexually and asexually. Most fungi are saprophytes. They secrete enzymes which digest the substrate and then absorb soluble nutrition thus produced. Scientists who study fungi are known as mycologist and the scientist discipline dealing with fungus is called mycology. The diseases caused by fungus in animal are known as mycoses. According to Whittaker classification, fungi are placed in the kingdom Fungi. There are six major groups as follows:

1. **Acrasiomycetes (cellular slime moulds):** These can be isolated from humus containing soils. The basic units of acrasiomycetes are necked, uninucleate, haploid, amoebae

like organisms. They move on solid medium with the help of pseudopodia, feed by phagocytosis of bacteria and multiply, e.g. *Dictyostelium mucoroides.*

2. **Myxomycetes (true slime moulds):** The spores liberated from the fruiting bodies germinate on moist surface and produce flagellate swarmers. They lose their flagella after some interval and enter amoeboid stage. At this stage, they may fuse with each other to form multinucleate plasmodia. This plasmodia give rise to fruiting bodies or sporangia containing unicellular spores.

3. **Phycomycetes (lower fungi):** It is large group of fungi with uniseptated and multinucleated vegetative bodies called Coenocytic thallus. They produce spores in sporangia. They are further divided into three classes:

   Chytridiomycetes: They can be parasites or saprophytes and are found on decaying plant material, microscopic animals, algae and water.

   Oomycetes: They are aquatic and terrestrial fungi that reproduce asexually.

   Zygomycetes: e.g. Rhizopus (bread mould), pilobolus, mucor.

4. **Ascomycetes (sac fungi):** They are higher fungi. They are characterized by a septated mycelium and formation of condiospores. Yeast belongs to protoascomycetes.

5. **Basidiomycetes,** e.g. mushrooms (club fungi)

6. **Deuteromycetes** (fungi imperfecti)

Fungal Disease

Mycosis of skin hair nails. It also infects plants and crop, e.g. *Tinea corporis* (ring worm) *Tinea capitis,* etc.

Yeast infection *Candida albicans*

Yeast is unicellular fungi that have a single nucleus. They reproduce either asexually by budding and transverse division or sexually through spore formation.

Medical Significance

Many of the human disease especially skin infections are associated with fungus. Tinea infection is widespread skin infection.

T. corporis : Ring worm infection

T. pedis   : Foot infection

T. barbae   : Beard infection

T. capitis   : Scalp infection

T. *cruris*   : Joint infection

Candida albicans is responsible for causing thrash, cystitis, endometritis and candidiasis. Fungus also attacks crops, garden plants and many wild plants.

Industrial Significance of Yeast

Yeast has been used in extensively in fermentation industry over the years. It is the main ingredient responsible for the rising of dough in the bakery industry. Many solvents and reagents like alcohol, acetic acid, isobutanol, lactic acid, butyric acid, acetone, formalin etc. can be prepared using different species of yeast. Yeast have also utility in preparation of sausage, wine, beer and cheese. Nucleic acids particularly RNA is obtained from *Candida utilis* and saccharomyces. These are used as a raw material in Biotechnology. β galactosidase is obtain from *S. fragilis* or *C. pseudotropicalis*. It is used to prepare lactose free milk products. Enzymes namely alcohol dehydrogenase, hexokinase, etc. are obtained from *Saccharomyces cerevisiae* which have extensive industrial utilization.

Nutrition of Fungi

Fungi grow best in dark, moist habitats but they are found wherever organic material is available. Most fungi are saprophytes; they get their nutrients from dead organic material. Fungi secrete hydrolytic enzyme that digest external substrates. Then they absorb the soluble products. They are chemoorganoheterotrophs and use organic material as a source of carbon, electrons and energy. Glycogen is primary stored carbohydrate in fungi. They are usually aerobic, some yeasts however are anaerobic and obtain energy by fermentation. Fungi can be cultivated in laboratory on sabouraud dextrose agar media. They require high sugar concentration and low pH.

Structure of Fungi

Fungal cells comprise of the elongated hyphae (Fig. 2.15) and are typically binucleate or multinucleate. One cell in the hyphae may be separated from another by a cross wall or septum. In some case like mastigomycota, there is presence of pseudo septa, i.e. septa is perforated to form sieve like structure. In basidiomycetes and deuteromycetes, the septum is more complex.

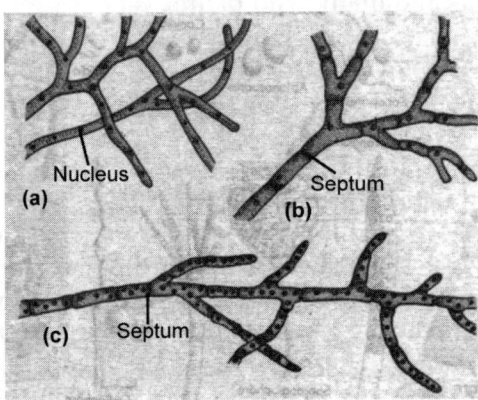

Fig. 2.15: Three types of hyphae (a) Nonseptate (coenocytic); (b) Septate with uninuleate cells; (c) Septate with multinucleate cells

The organism like yeast exists as unicellular cells and generally reproduces by budding. The fungal cell walls are comparatively thin about 0.2 μ thick. Its composition varies from species to species. It may contain fungal cellulose, pectose, chitin or callose. Protoplast consists of plasma membrane, cytoplasm, nucleus and other eukaryotic cell components.

Fungi lack chlorophyll and are non-photosynthetic. They do not have specialized tissue like higher organisms but are rather filamentous in nature. During asexual reproduction fungus produce spores which differ from species to species. Spores are located in the upper ends of the aerial hyphae (Fig. 2.16).

Importance of Fungi

It is used in many industries involving fermentation, e.g. For manufacturing of wine, beer, bread, cheese, etc. It is also

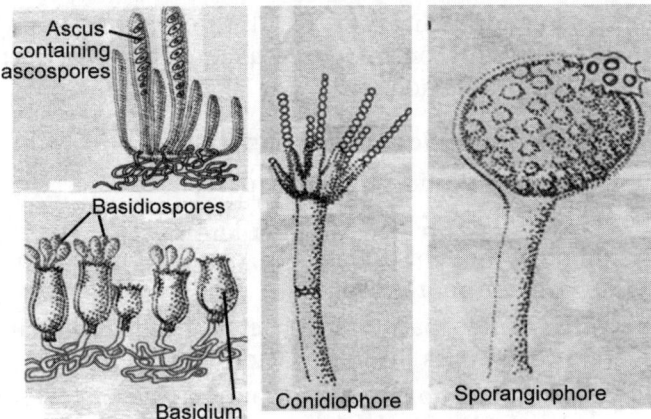

Fig. 2.16: Spore types in fungi

used in biotransformation reaction because many fungi produce enzyme useful for biotransformation reaction, e.g. manufacturing of corticosteroids. Various enzymes like lipase, amylase, protease, etc. and vitamins like B_1, B_2, B_6 and biotin are manufactured by fungi, e.g. *Aspergillus* species produce protease invertase.

VII. RICKETTSIA

They are intracellular parasites. They are usually gram-negative and multiply only within the host cells by binary fission. They cause disease via insect vectors. They are smaller in size. They occur singly, in pairs or occasionally in strands.

They multiply only within certain cells of susceptible hosts. Acute infections are characterized clinically by fever, headache and rashes. The organisms occur under natural conditions in lice, fleas, ticks and mites. These arthropods are the primary means of transmission to man. Rickettsia are easily grown in large numbers in the yolk sac of chick embryo and cell cultures. Penetration into the host cells requires the expenditure of energy. The Rickettsial cell wall is like gram-negative bacteria, it contains both peptidoglycan and lipopolysaccharide.

Pathogenesis

Rickettsial infections in humans begin in the vascular systems following the bite of infected arthropod. The microorganism proliferates in endothelial cells. Death results from damage to endothelial cells with consequence leakage of plasma, decrease in blood volume and shock.

General Characteristics of Rickettsia

1. They are prokaryotic, obligatory parasites.
2. These are gram-negative bacteria.
3. The shape of these bacteria is rod, coccoid or pleomorphic.
4. They are non-motile
5. They are smaller than typical bacterial cells. Like viruses, several species pass through bacteriological filters.
6. They reproduce by binary fission and replicate in cytoplasm and nucleus of host cells.
7. Acute infection is characterized by fever, headache and rash.
8. They are sensitive to the wide spectrum of antibiotics, e.g. tetracycline, chloramphenicol.
9. Although metabolic machinery is present, but it is defective. It lacks the ability to synthesize important enzymes rendering the Rickettsia to depend on host for energy metabolism.
10. Cultivation is possible on small rodents or on yolk sac of chick embryo.

Examples of Human Rickettsial Infections

Epidemic typhus by *R. prowazekii* had resulted in approximately three million deaths in both World War I and II. As it is transmitted by *louse*, it is generally a result of overcrowding and poor hygiene (Table 2.1).

Table 2.1: Examples of human Rickettsial infections

Infections	Causative agent	Arthropod vector
Epidemic typhus fever	*Rickettsia prowazekii*	Louse
Endemic typhus	*Rickettsia typhi*	–
Rocky mountain spotted fever	*R. rickettsiae*	Tick
Q-fever	*Coxiella burnetii*	–

Q-fever is generally acquired by inhalation of contaminated aerosols or ingestion of contaminated milk or food.

Growth and Metabolism

- They are grown in large number in yolk sac of the chick embryo and cell culture.
- Rickettsia multiplies by transverse binary fission, within the vesicles in the cytoplasm of host cell, which protect them from lysosomal degradation.
- The generation time is much longer than that of most bacteria.
- Rickettsias are released by host cell lysis or via a vesicle in the host cell membrane.

VIII. SPIROCHETES

Spira means coil (curved) and *chaete* meaning cork shaped (hair). Spirochetes are slender, flexible, helically coiled, unicellular organism. The name itself suggests that they are of spiral structure. They differ from bacteria's and viruses in structure, as they are like cork screw spiral structure. Size varies from 0.3 to 1.5 μm width, 7 to 500 μm length. The body of spirochetes consists of axial filament and cytoplasm found spirally around the cytoplasm (Fig. 2.17).

Spirochetes have a three-layer outer membrane. They do not possess cell wall characteristics of bacteria. Very delicate terminal filaments resembling flagella have been viewed in some species. Spirochetes are actively mobile due to the

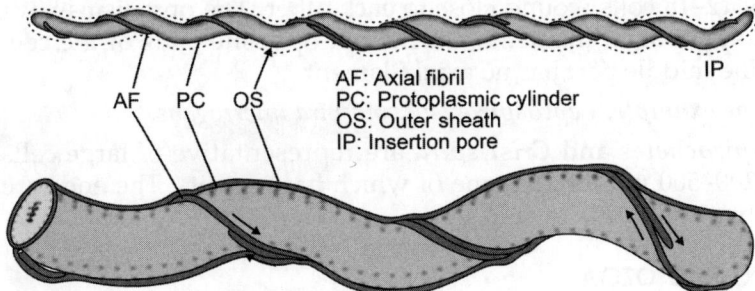

AF: Axial fibril
PC: Protoplasmic cylinder
OS: Outer sheath
IP: Insertion pore

AF PC OS

IP

Fig. 2.17: Basic anatomical components of spirochetes as interpreted from electron micrographs

distinct flexibility of their body. The second type of movement is in rotating manner, performed axially, a translational movement forward and backwards. It also performs bending movement. They are motile because of intrinsic active bending movement.

Classification

Order: Spirochaetales

Family: Spirochaetaceae

Mainly spirochete lives on dead substrates in foul water and in the guts of cold blooded animals.

Genera:

1. Borrelia
2. Treponema
3. Leptospira
4. Spirochaeta
5. Cristispira

Borrelia: They have large obtuse angled irregular spirals numbering from 3–10. *B. hispania* causing relapsing fever and *B. persica* are passed into human through lice and ticks.

Treponema (Means—thread—like): Treponema exhibits thin flexible cells with 6–14 twists. The microorganisms do not appear to have visible axial filament or an axial crest. The end of Treponema is either tapered or round. Some species have thread on the poles, e.g. *Treponema pallidum.*

Leptospira (Leptos-Thin and Spira-Coiled): Organisms of this genus are characterized by very thin cell structure consisting of 12–18 coils wound close to each other. The organisms have a spore axial filaments attached at opposite ends of the cell. The middle part has no axial filament.

For example, Leptospirosis: Leptospira interrogans.

Spirochetes and *Cristispira* are representative of large cells (200–500 μm long). Some of which have crypts. The ends are sharp or blunt.

IX. PROTOZOA

They are unicellular, eukaryotic, chemoheterotrophs found in the soil, water or as normal microbiota in animals. The name is derived from two Greek words "proton" (first) and "zoon" (animal). Asexual reproduction is by fusion or budding while sexual reproduction is by conjugation. Some of them produce cyst for protection during adverse environmental conditions. The cyst permits the organism to survive when food, moisture or oxygen supply are not sufficient.

Nutrition

Mostly aerobic heterotrophs ciliates take food by moving cilia towards the mouth like opening called cytostome. Amoeba engulfs food by surrounding it with pseudopods and phagocytizing it. Taxonomy is based on type of movement, reproduction and development cycle. Medically important phylums are as follows:

Class 1: *Mastigophora (Flagellates)*

One or more flagella typically present in trophozoites.

1. **Family:** Trypanosomatidae

   Genus: *Trypanosomes*

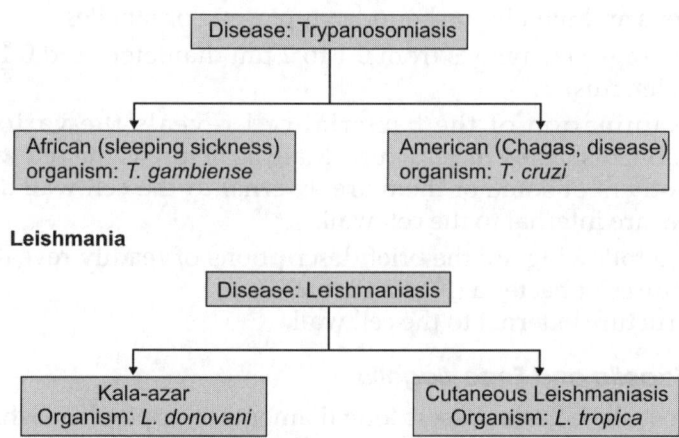

2. **Family:** Distomatidae

   Giardia lamblia cause diarrhea in children and Lambliasis is caused by *L. intestinalis*.

3. **Family:** Trichomonadidae

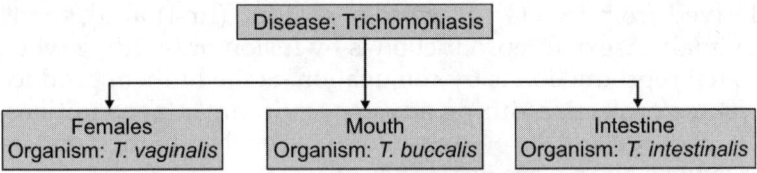

Class 2: **Lobosea**

Family: Endamoebidae, e.g. *Entamoeba histolytica* causes Amoebiasis

Class 3: *Sporozoa*

a. **Genus:** *Plasmodium*

Plasmodium vivax, Plasmodium ovale, Plasmodium malariae and Plasmodium falciparum causes malaria

b. **Toxoplasma:** *T. gondii* causes toxoplasmosis

X. STRUCTURE OF BACTERIAL CELL

Bacterial cell is typical prokaryotic cell which is the simplest and first type of cells to evolve about 4.5 billion years ago. They have a nuclear body (nucleoid), i.e. there is absence of enveloped nucleus and membrane bound cytoplasmic organelles.

Average size ranges from 0.1 to 2 µm diameters and 0.1 to 8 µm lengths.

Examination of the bacterial cell reveals the various components inside its structure. Main structure is the cell wall and others of some of them are external to the cell wall and others are internal to the cell wall.

The following are the brief descriptions of readily revealed structures of bacteria (Figs 2.18 to 2.20).

Structure external to the cell wall.

1. Flagella and Endo-flagella

Almost all bacteria possess long filamentous appendage which protrudes out from the cell wall and are responsible for swimming motility, this is called *Flagella*.

Size

The length of flagellum is approximately 70 µm which is several times larger than the bacterial cell itself. The diameter

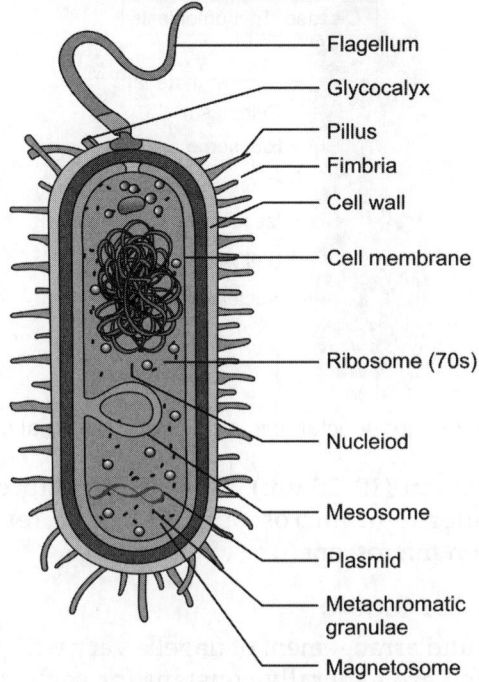

Fig. 2.18: Ultrastructure of typical bacterial cell

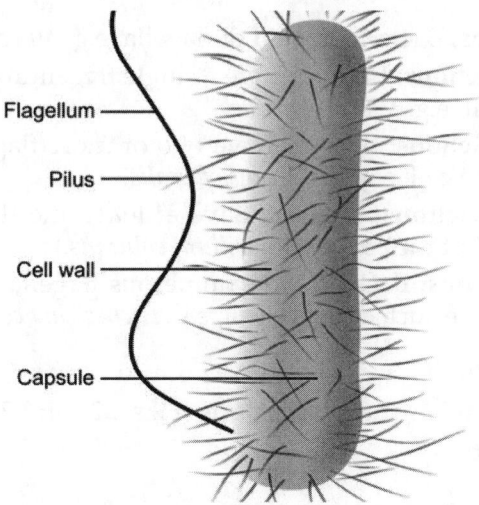

Fig. 2.19: Major structure external to the bacterial cell wall

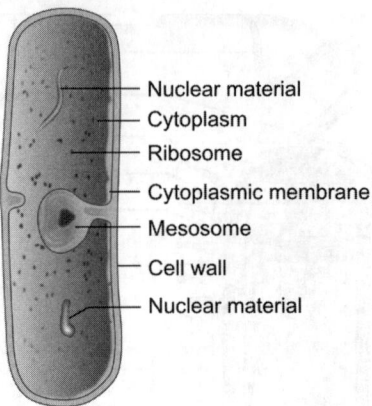

- Nuclear material
- Cytoplasm
- Ribosome
- Cytoplasmic membrane
- Mesosome
- Cell wall
- Nuclear material

Fig. 2.20: Major structures internal to the bacterial cell wall

is 0.01 to 0.02 μm (10–20 nm). This size structure cannot be revealed under light microscope but can be revealed only under electron microscope.

Arrangement of flagella

The number and arrangement of flagella vary with varying the bacteria. They are generally constant for each species. The arrangement pattern of flagella in different bacteria is as follows:

1. **Atrichous:** Bacteria devoid of flagella, e.g. all *cocci.*
2. **Monotrichous:** Bacteria have a single flagellum at one end of the cell, e.g. *Vibrio cholerae.*
3. **Lophotrichous:** Bacteria have two or more flagella at one end of the cell, e.g. *Alcaligenes faecalis.*
4. **Amphitrichous:** Bacteria have at least one flagellum at each end of the cell, e.g. *Spirillum volutans.*
5. **Peritrichous:** Bacteria have numerous flagella distributed all over the surface of the cell, e.g. *Escherichia coli.*

Ultrastructure

The flagellum has three basic parts (Figs 2.21 and 2.22):

1. Filament
2. Hook
3. Basal body

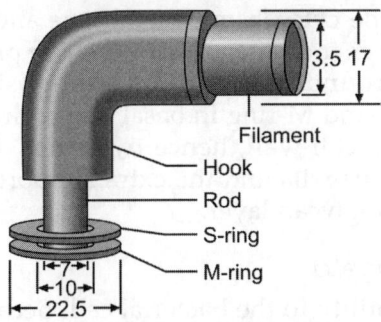

Fig. 2.21: Ultrastructure of flagella (gram-positive bacteria)

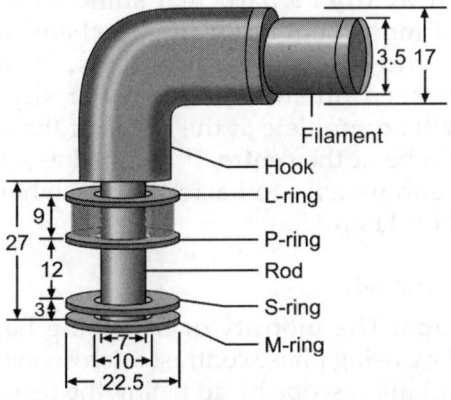

Fig. 2.22: Ultrastructure of flagella (gram-negative bacteria)

1. **Filament:** It is the outermost region which protrudes out of the cell surface. It is thin and cylindrical and has a constant diameter. It contains protein which is made up of monomers called '*Flagellin*' with molecular weight ranging between 20,000 and 40,000 Daltons.

2. **Hook:** The curved part which joins the filaments with basal body is Hook. The filament is attached to a slightly wider Hook. It is made up of proteins.

3. **Basal body:** It is composed of a small central rod which is inserted into a series of rings. Gram-negative bacteria contain four rings, i.e. L-ring, P-ring, S-ring, and M-ring. The L-ring is contained in lipopolysaccharide layer of outer membrane, P-ring in peptidoglycan layer, S-ring is

just above the cytoplasmic membrane and M-ring within cytoplasmic membrane. These rings are placed one above the other around central rod. Gram-positive organisms have only S-and M-ring in basal body. Gram-positive cell have a thick cell wall, hence two rings are sufficient to support the flagella and the extra support is provided by thick peptidoglycan layer.

Functions of flagella

It offers the motility to the bacterial cell. Because of motility, the bacterium moves towards favorable environment or away from adverse one. The movement of a bacterium towards or away from a particular stimulus is called Taxis. The bacterial movement according to chemical stimulus is Chemotaxis and to light is Phototaxis. If suspension of bacteria is placed on slide under cover slip, the aerobic organisms will accumulate at the edges of the cover slip and anaerobic will be at the centre. It is called aerotaxis. Flagella also impart antigenicity to bacterial cell, where filament is associated with H-antigen.

Detection of motility

1. **Microscope:** The motility of the living bacteria can be observed by using phase contrast microscope and also with compound microscope by adjusting the proper contrast.

2. **On the culture medium:** On the semisolid medium, motile microbes can swim throughout the plate. The presence of turbidity throughout the plate is a positive test for the presence of motility.

3. **Electron microscope:** The high magnification and resolution of the electron microscope with common staining will evaluate the motility easily.

4. **Staining:** Flagella can be coated with stains like basic fuchsine, the dye will be bound to the structure will provide extra width to the structure which makes them visible under light microscope.

5. **Antibody stains:** By attaching a fluorescent dye to the antibody and using a fluorescence microscope will detect the flagellin.

Mechanism of flagellar movement

Flagella are semi-rigid, helical rotors which rotate either clockwise or anticlockwise around its long axis. Movement is enhanced by relative rotation of S and M rings. In gram-positive motile bacteria only S and M rings are present. It indicates that only these rings are involved in motility. L and P rings give mechanical support because the gram-negative cell wall is thin.

Endoflagellum (axial filament)

The flagella present within the outer sheath will arise at one end and present spirally around the cell, which is called as endoflagellum or axial filament. Rotation of filament leads to movement of bacteria. This rotation is just like corkscrew motion. Endoflagella are generally detected in Spirochetes, e.g. *Treponema pallidum*.

2. Pili (Latin—Hairs)

Pili are longer than the fimbriae and they are only few in numbers per cell (one or two per cell).

There are two basic functions for pili, i.e. gene transfer and attachment.

They are known to be receptors for the certain bacterial viruses. The pili is also referred as *sex pili*. The sex pilus (or F pilus) is involved in conjugation process in certain bacteria, where, the donor bacteria attaches to a recipient via the sex pilus. Then the copy of small fragment of the donor bacteria's genome will pass through the sex pilus into the recipient. The drug resistance in many different species of bacteria spreads by this mechanism.

3. Fimbriae (Latin—Fringes)

Fimbriae are shorter and straighter than the flagella and are more numerous. The numbers of fimbriae ranges from few to hundreds. Not all the bacteria synthesize them. Fimbriae do not play any role in motility, but they are thought to be important in the attachment to the surfaces. The microbe will become much more virulent when it is able to synthesize fimbriae.

4. Glycocalyx

An extracellular, slimy or mucilaginous layer external to the cell wall that is formed by several bacteria is called as *glycocalyx*.

Glycocalyx means *'sugar-coat'*. However, this structure is not essential for viability of the cell. The glycocalyx is well organized and firmly attached to the cell wall which is called as *Capsule*. While, the glycocalyx, unorganized and loosely attached to the cell wall is called as *Slime layer* (Fig. 2.23).

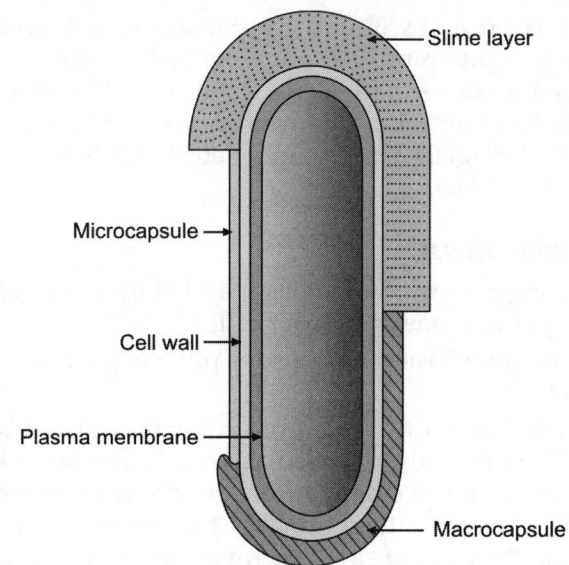

Fig. 2.23: Glycocalyx

Size

Capsule layer may be thin or thick and it differs from species to species. The thin layer having size less than 0.2 µm is called as microcapsule, such structure is not detected by light microscope. The thick layer having size more than 0.2 µm up to 10 µm is called as *macrocapsule.*

Composition of capsule

Water is the chief component of bacterial capsule (98%). The most common organic constituent of bacterial capsule is *polysaccharide*. It may contain homopolysaccharide or heteropolysaccharide. Several bacteria also contain peptides/proteins in the capsule, e.g. the capsule of *Bacillus anthracis* is composed of γ-glutamyl polypeptide.

Functions of capsule

The exact function of the capsule is not properly understood. However, capsule may play an important role in following:

1. Protection from desiccation
2. Protection from bacteriophages
3. Antiphagocytic factor
4. Promotes stability by preventing cell aggregate formation.

Detection of capsule

It can be detected by staining techniques like manual method, Hiss method. (Detailed description is given in this chapter, under topic capsule staining.) It can also be detected by Quellungs reaction.

Cell wall

Just outside the plasma membrane, a complex semi-rigid structure which determines the shape of bacteria is referred to as cell wall. Cell wall is the most important structure of the bacteria because the most bacteria cannot live without it. Exceptionally, *Mycoplasma* species and several archaea do not have cell wall at all. Thus the presence of the cell wall is a unique characteristic of the bacteria; that is two types of cell wall are detected in bacteria, i.e. gram-positive and gram-negative types of cell wall. This is due to different chemical composition of the cell wall which gives the differential staining response. Gram-positive and gram-negative cells have one thing common in them, i.e. unique bacteria and it is the presence of peptidoglycan.

Structure of gram-positive cell Wall

The size of gram-positive cell wall ranges from 20 to 80 nm. It constituted of one thick layer. The cell wall of the gram-positive bacteria is stronger than the gram-negative cell wall as the gram-positive cell wall contains peptidoglycan and teichoic acid (Fig. 2.24).

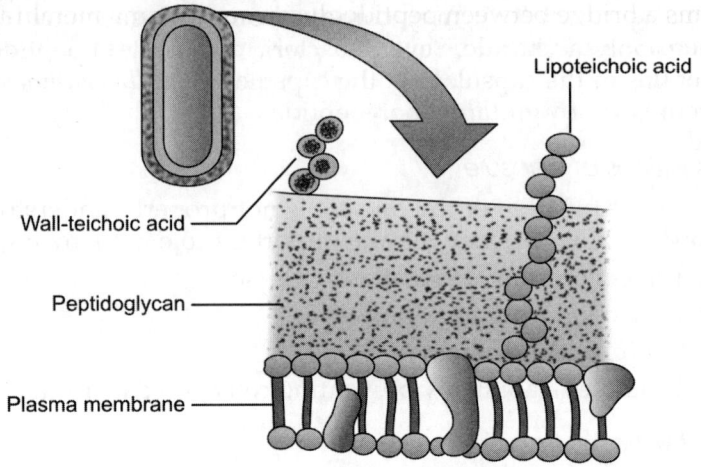

Fig. 2.24: Ultrastructure of gram-positive cell wall

Peptidoglycan

It is a thick rigid layer and is composed of a two sugars, i.e. N-acetyl glucosamine (NAG) and N-acetyl muramic (NAM) acid. These sugars are covalently bound by β-(1–4) linkage. Generally, a side chain of 4-amino acids is attached to NAM. The amino acid composition of side chain varies from species to species. The most commonly found 4-amino acids are L-alanine, D-alanine, D-glutamic acid and diaminopimelic acid (DPA). Generally, the living system is made up of L-isomer. It is important to note that both the gram-positive and gram-negative bacteria possess peptidoglycans in their cell wall. In gram-positive bacteria, the peptide chains are highly crosslinked (e.g. *Staphylococcus aureus*) but in gram-negative bacteria the peptide chains are partially crosslinked.

Teichoic acid

It is also an important component in the gram-positive cell wall. It is a polymer of glycerol or ribitol joined by phosphate groups. The teichoic acids possess a strong negative charge and they are highly antigenic. These are generally absent in gram-negative bacteria. They are present in two forms, i.e. lipoteichoic acid and wall-teichoic acid. The lipoteichoic acid forms a bridge between peptidoglycan and plasma membrane whereas, wall-teichoic acid is present within the peptidoglycan layer (Fig. 2.25). Lipoteichoic acids are polymers of amphiphilic glycophosphates with the lipophilic glycolipid. Lipoteichoic acids are antigenic and cytotoxic in nature, e.g. *Streptococcus pyogenes*.

Structure of gram-negative cell wall

The cell wall of gram-negative bacteria is having more complicated structure. It is made up of two separate layers.

1. The outer membrane
2. The thin layer of peptidoglycan

1. **The outer membrane:** The thickness of outer membrane is 7–8 nm. The outer membrane is a lipid bilayer which is somewhat similar to the plasma membrane. It contains the lipopolysaccharide, proteins and also lipids.

   a. **Lipopolysaccharide (LPS):** It is composed of two parts, lipid A and the polysaccharide chain. Lipopolysaccharide contains the negative charge and thus repels the hydrophobic molecules. There are some examples of gram-negative species that have found in the gut of mammals where, LPS will repel the fat solubilizing

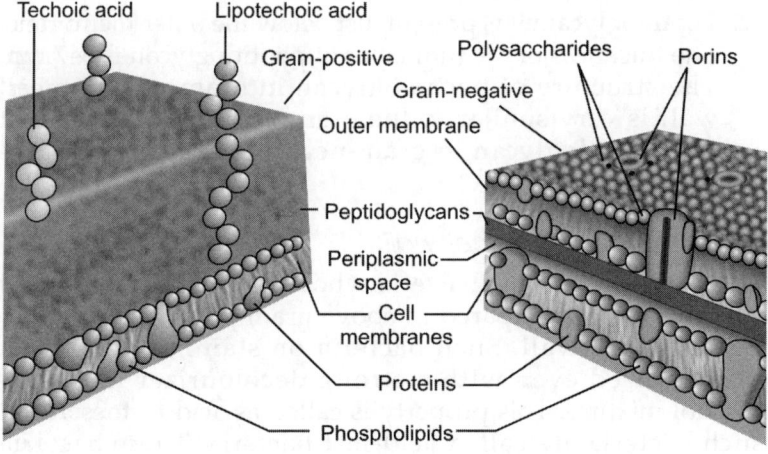

Fig. 2.25: Ultrastructure of gram-negative cell wall

molecules like bile (generally secreted by gallbladder). The O-antigen is associated with LPS. The characteristic feature found in gram-negative bacteria is the presence of complex macromolecular LPS. These are also called endotoxins which are cell bound and heat stable toxins. The endotoxin plays an important role in the pathogenesis of many gram-negative bacterial infections.

b. **Protein:** There are fewer types but many numbers of proteins which are found in outer membrane as compared to cytoplasmic membrane. Porins are specialized proteins which forms the pores in the outer membrane. These pores are wide enough so that they allow the passage of small molecules like peptides, nucleotide, amino acid, vitamin B_{12} and iron. This passage allows the migration of the molecules into the periplasmic space for transport across the cytoplasmic membrane.

Larger or hydrophobic molecules cannot penetrate the outer membrane.

c. **Periplasmic space:** It is the space between the outer membrane and plasma membrane which will varies from 1 to 71 nm, e.g. hydrolytic enzymes, binding proteins, etc. The fluid present in this space is called periplasm. The fluid includes several proteins, which will transport the nutrients into the cell.

2. **Peptidoglycan:** It is present just below the outer membrane. The thickness of the thin layer of peptidoglycan is 3–7 nm. The structure of peptidoglycan in gram-negative cell wall is very similar to the gram-positive cell wall but the peptidoglycan in gram-negative cell contains less crosslinking.

Structure of acid-fast cell wall

There are again some bacteria whose cell wall has different composition as compared to above gram-positive and gram-negative cell wall. Such bacteria on staining do not get decolourised even with a strong decolourizer like acid-alcohol mixture. This property is called as acid-fastness. And such bacteria are called acid-fast bacteria. These bacteria contain mycolic acid and other waxy material along with peptidoglycan in their cell wall, e.g. *Mycobacterium* species and several Actinomycetes.

Functions of the cell wall

1. It determines the shape of bacteria.
2. It provides strength to bacterial cell.
3. It protects the cell from the toxic substances.
4. It confers the pathogenicity to several pathogens.
5. In the cell wall of gram-negative bacteria, the outer membrane is barrier to several harmful substances like antibiotics, enzymes and heavy metals.

Comparison of cell walls of gram-positive and gram-negative bacteria

Comparison of gram-positive and gram-negative cell walls is shown in Table 2.2.

Table 2.2: Comparison of gram-positive and gram-negative bacterial cell wall

Component	Gram-positive	Gram-negative
Thickness	Thick (20–25 nm)	Thin (10–15 nm)
Peptidoglycan	More (50–90%)	Less/95–10%
Teichoic acid	Present	Absent
Polysaccharide	Present	Absent
Lipids	Less or absent	More
Cell wall	Simple	Complex
Outer membrane and periplasmic space	Absent	Present
Effect of lysozyme	Easily destroyed	Resistant
Type of amino acids	Few	Several
Susceptibility to streptomycin and tetracycline	Slight	Marked
Susceptibility to penicillin and sulfonamides	Marked	Much less
Examples	*Bacillus anthracis, Clostridium tetani, S. aureus*	*Escherichia coli, Salmonella typhi, Vibrio cholerae*

Structure internal to the cell wall

1. Plasma membrane

It is the thin structure made up of proteins and phospholipids, which encloses the cytoplasm and controls the transport across the cell. It is called as cytoplasmic, protoplast or inner membrane. It is a sheet like structure. The thickness of the bacterial plasma membrane ranges between 5–10 nm. Plasma membrane contains lipids, proteins and trace amount of carbohydrates (Fig. 2.26). As compared to eukaryotic cell, the bacterial plasma membrane contains the high portion of proteins. The ratio of protein is to phospholipid in the bacterial plasma membrane is 3:1. The proteins present in the membrane serves as channels, receptors and enzymes. The lipid bilayer creates the suitable environment for orientation and activity of proteins. The lipids and proteins are held together by non-covalent bond. The plasma membrane is electrically polarized. The membrane potential plays an important role in transport, biosynthesis, energy conversion, etc.

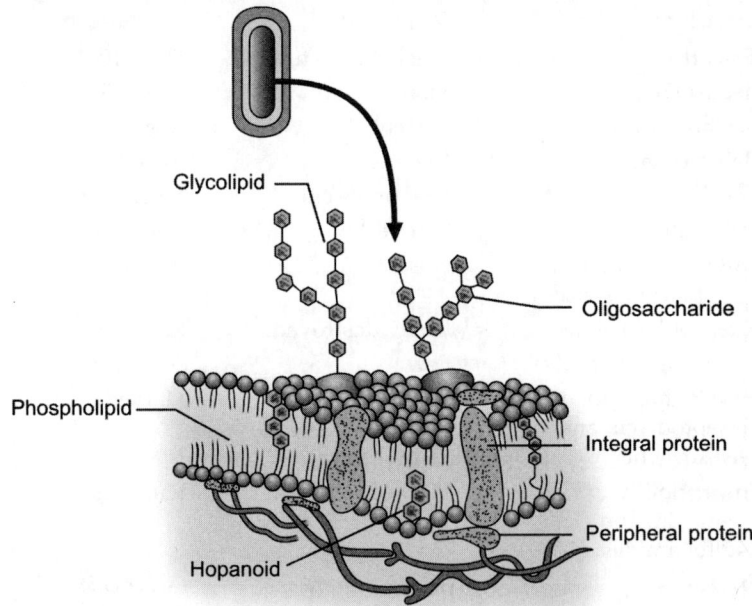

Fig. 2.26: Structure of plasma membrane

2. Mesosomes

Inner folding of the cell membrane is called as mesosome. It provides extra space for enzymatic reaction. The mesosomes are detected in both the gram-positive and gram-negative bacteria but are more prominent in gram-positive bacteria.

Function

It involves in the formation of cell wall during the cell division. It provides the extra space for enzymatic reaction. It plays an important role in DNA replication and proper distribution of cytoplasm in daughter cell.

3. Ribosomes

The granular small bodies made up of protein and r-RNA is called as Ribosomes. They are involved in protein synthesis. It gives the typical granular appearance to the cytoplasm. The unit of which is given by 'S'. There are 70S in bacteria. The 70S ribosome is actually made up of two subunits 50S and 30S.

Svedberg unit

It is the unit of sedimentation coefficient and denoted by 'S'. It is used to measure the sedimentation velocity, i.e. how faster particle sediment in ultracentrifuge. The dimension of ribosome is 14–15 × 20 nm and molecular weight is about 2.7 million. The bacterial cell contains 5000–50000 ribosomes.

Composition

Ribosomes are RNA containing bodies. They are composed of protein and RNA. The specialized type of RNA is present which is called as rRNA (ribosomal RNA)

Function

It is actively involved in protein synthesis. Thus gives catalytic role (enzyme). It is also important for viability of cell and metabolic activity.

4. Cell inclusions

It is the reserved component which is present within the bacterial cytoplasm that is called as cell inclusions. The cell inclusions are helpful in identification of the bacteria. Many cell inclusions can be seen in bacteria which are summarized as follows (Table 2.3):

Table 2.3: Cell inclusion complex composition and significance

Cell inclusion	Composition	Significance
Metachromatic granule/volutin/ Babes granule	Polyphosphate granules	Reserve the source of phosphate
Lipid granules	Polyhydroxy butyrate granules	Reserve source of lipid
Carboxysomes	Ribulose 1,5 diphosphate carboxylase	Important enzyme for photosynthesis
Gas vacuoles	Gas (e.g. CO_2, H_2S)	Maintain buoyancy to get oxygen, light and nutrients
Magnetosome	Iron oxide (Fe_3O_4)	Direct the cell to proper environment

5. Nucleoid

The nuclear area is called nucleoid. There is not typical nucleus present in the bacterial cell. It contains single circular double stranded DNA which is known as bacterial chromosome or bacterial genome. The bacterial DNA is attached to plasma membrane at several points. It is lack of histone protein but the function of histone can be fulfilled by low molecular weight polyamines and magnesium ions. Nucleoid occupies 29% of cell volume.

Function

DNA is the hereditary material which controls nearly all functions of the cell.

Detection of nuclear material

Bacterial chromosome is visible under light microscope after staining by Feulgen stain.

6. Plasmid

In bacterial cells, besides one main chromosome, some other pieces of genetic material is observed. These other pieces of DNA are called as *plasmid*. The plasmids are extra-chromosomal pieces of DNA. Plasmids are similar to chromosome but are smaller in size. The size of the plasmids ranges from 1–200 kb (kilobases); whereas size of chromosome is about 4000kb. The plasmids are circular DNA; linear plasmids also exist in few species. The number of a plasmid in a cell varies from 1 to 700.

Function

Plasmids are not essential though they may play important role for the bacteria.

1. **Antibiotic resistance:** Some plasmids may code for the proteins and degrades the antibiotic. Thus they can produce resistance.

2. **Virulence factor,** e.g. *E. coli plasmic Ent P307* may codes for an enterotoxin and hence, makes the *E. coli* pathogenic.

3. **Conjugation:** Conjugative plasmids allow the exchange of DNA between the bacterial cells. Plasmids are also important in recombinant DNA technology.

7. Endospore

Under certain conditions of limited supply of nutrients or water, some bacteria may produce specialized 'resting' cell bodies which are called as *endospore* (Fig. 2.27). Endospores are detected in gram-positive bacteria and gram-negative species also. These bacteria forms endospore like structure and thus resist heat and chemicals. Two main genera of endospore forming bacteria are *Bacillus* and *Clostridium*. Other spore forming genera includes the *Sporolactobacillus, Sporosarcina, Desulfotomaculum* and *Actinomycetes*.

Position

They may be oval, ellipsoid or spherical in shape and may be present at central, sub terminal or terminal position.

Ultrastructure

It consists of protoplast or core, spore integument or envelope. The protoplast contains DNA and some components of protein synthesis such as ribosomes, t-RNAs and enzymes, there is no m-RNA is detected. From the inner to the outer side, the spore envelope contains inner membrane, the cortex, the outer membrane and the spore coat. In some species, an additional

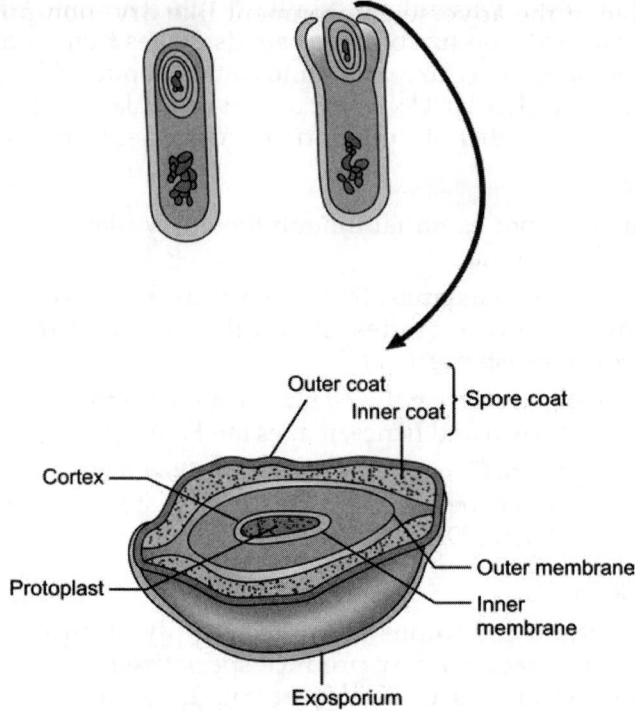

Fig. 2.27: Ultrastructure of endospore

covering called exosporium is present around the spore coat (e.g. *Bacillus cereus*). The exosporium contains polysaccharide, protein membrane, and small amount of lipids, which loosely covers the spores. The multi-laminated cortex develops between the inner and outer membrane which consist of peptidoglycan and important component dipicolinic acid (2, 6 pyridine carboxylic acid). It also contains large amounts of calcium ions, mainly in the form of calcium dipicolinate. The spore coat is formed outside the outer membrane which is made up of the keratin like protein. The spore coat proteins contain abundance of cysteine and hydrophobic amino acids. The spore coat confers the resistance to spore from the chemicals.

Importance of endospore

They are heat and chemical resistant, also resistant to drying, freezing and radiation. Thus the main ecological role is to survive in the adverse environment like dry, non-nutrient environment.

Table 2.4 describes the difference between vegetative cell and endospore.

Table 2.4: Difference between vegetative cell and endospore

Vegetative cell	Endospore
It is readily stained by ordinary stains. Usually stains gram-positive organisms	It does not readily stained by ordinary stains
Sensitive to various physical and chemical agents such as heat radiation, disinfectant and antibiotic	Resistance to various physical and chemical agents such as heat radiation, disinfectant and antibiotic
Contains relatively low sulfur containing amino acids	Contains high sulfur containing amino acid and calcium
Calcium ions and dipicolinic acid are absent	Calcium ions and dipicolinic acid are present
Metabolically active	Metabolically inactive (activities are negligible)

XI. NUTRITIONAL REQUIREMENTS OF BACTERIA

A. Nutrition Required for the Growth

1. Source of Energy

Some microbes rely on the chemical compounds for their energy and known as chemotrophs, e.g. *Escherichia coli*. Some microbes utilizes radiant energy (sunlight) and are called phototrophs, e.g. *Rhodospirillum rubrum*.

2. Source of Electrons

All the microbes require electrons for their metabolism. Some organisms can use reduced inorganic compounds as electron donors and are termed as lithotrophs (some may be chemolithotrophs and others may be photolithotrophs), e.g. *Pseudomonas pseudoflava*. Some organism uses organic compound as an electron donor and are called as organotrophs (some may be chemoorganotrophs and others photoorganotrophs), e.g. *Escherichia coli*.

3. Source of Carbon

All microorganisms require carbon for synthesizing cell components. some microorganism use carbon dioxide as their major or even sole, source of carbon and are termed as autotrophs, e.g. *Chromatium okenii*. Some microbes require organic compound as their carbon source are termed as heterotrophs, e.g. *Escherichia coli*

4. Nitrogen

Bacteria use nitrogen from the atmosphere or from the inorganic compounds such as nitrates, nitrites, ammonium salts or organic compounds such as amino acids. Nitrogen is a major component of protein and nucleic acids.

5. Sulphur

Many bacterial species use sulphur from organic sulphur compounds, inorganic sulphur compounds and elemental sulphur. It is needed for synthesis of amino acids.

6. Phosphorus

Phosphorus, usually supplied in the form of phosphate is an essential component of nucleotides, nucleic acids, phospholipids, etc.

7. Mineral Salts

Bacteria require salts, particularly the anions such as phosphate and sulphate and the cations as sodium, potassium, magnesium, iron and calcium. These are normally present in the natural environments or may be added in culture media.

8. Vitamins and Vitamin-like Compounds

Some bacterial species require organic compounds in minute quantities for growth. These are known as growth factor or bacterial vitamins. Some bacteria are capable of synthesizing their entire requirement of vitamins from culture medium. Some other species cannot synthesize the vitamins from media and do not show growth in the absence of vitamins. Hence, for the growth of these species, vitamins are added in the culture media.

9. Water

It is the major essential nutrient as it accounts for about 80 to 90% of the total weight of cells. Water is a highly polar compound and it contains micronutrients and trace elements which are required for the growth of bacteria.

B. Nutrient Media Required for the Growth

Media are an artificially prepared mixture of various nutrients for the growth and multiplication of microorganism. A wide variety of culture media are employed by a microbiologist for the isolation, growth, purification, maintenance and identification of microorganisms. A culture media must supply suitable carbon, nitrogen, energy sources and other nutrients. Nutrient agar is a common laboratory medium used for growth of may bacterial species. It is notable that not a single media is suitable for growth of all microorganisms.

Common ingredients of media

1. **Water:** Tap, pure or distilled water may be used for the preparation of culture media by dissolving various organic and inorganic compounds. In the protoplasm of the cell, 70–80% water is present and it acts as a vehicle for the flow of nutrients. All enzymatically controlled chemical reactions occur within the cell in the presence of water.

2. **Peptone:** It is a complex mixture of partially digested proteins obtained from lean meat, heart muscle, casein, fibrin, soya meal, etc. The important constituents are proteases, amino acids, inorganic salts which include phosphates, potassium and magnesium and growth factors including nicotinic acid and riboflavin. Peptones mainly supply nitrogenous material and also act as a buffer. Peptone is stored in the tightly closed container because it is hygroscopic and becomes sticky when exposed to air.

3. **Yeast extract:** Yeast extract is prepared from the cells of baker's yeast or *Saccharomyces*.

   It contains carbohydrates, amino acids, growth factors (vitamin B group) and inorganic salts. Yeast extract is used mainly as a source of vitamins and may be substituted for meat extract.

4. **Meat extract:** It is prepared from fresh lean meat by hot water extraction process. It contains gelatin, peptones, proteoses, amino acids, creatine, creatinine, purines, mineral salts, carbohydrates and growth factors include thiamine, nicotinic acid, riboflavin, pyridoxine and pantothenic acid.

5. **Agar:** Agar is a long chain polysaccharide obtained from seaweeds algae. These algae which give agar are called *Agarophytes*. Agar is a mixture of two polysaccharides such as agarose (70%) and agaropectin (30%). It also contains calcium, chloride, magnesium, sulphate, iron, etc. Agar or agar-agar is now commonly used for the preparation of solid media.

Types of culture media

Culture media may be classified in different ways:

a. Depending on physical state (media consistency)
   i. Solid media (1.5–2.5% agar), e.g. nutrient agar.
   ii. Semisolid media (0.2–0.5% agar), e.g. nutrient broth containing 0.5% agar.
   iii. Liquid media (absence of agar), e.g. fluid thioglycollate broth.

b. Depending on oxygen requirement
   i. Aerobic media, e.g. MacConkey's broth
   ii. Anaerobic media, e.g. Robertson's cooked meat medium

c. Depending on chemical composition
   i. Simple or basal media
   ii. Synthetic or defined media
   iii. Non-synthetic or undefined or complex media.

d. Depending on functional type
   i. Enriched media
   ii. Enrichment media
   iii. Selective media
   iv. Indicator media
   v. Differential media
   vi. Sugar media
   vii. Transport media

viii. Assay media

ix. Storage media.

1. Simple or Basal Media

These media includes peptone water and nutrient broths which form the basis of most media used in the study of common bacteria. Addition of 2% agar to nutrient broth forms a nutrient agar medium which is a solid basal medium.

2. Complex or Non-synthetic or Undefined Media

They usually contain complex biological material such as blood or milk or yeast extract or beef extract. The exact chemical composition of this media is not known but it provides all the growth factors for the cultivation of unknown bacteria.

3. Synthetic or Defined Media

These media are prepared from pure chemical substances and the exact composition of the medium is known. These media are used for research purposes as well as metabolic studies of different microorganisms.

4. Enriched Media

These are prepared for fastidious microorganisms by addition of substances such as blood, serum and egg to basal medium, e.g. Blood agar (*Streptococcus*), chocolate agar (*Neisseria*).

5. Enrichment Media

When a specific substance is added in a liquid medium which inhibits the growth of unwanted bacteria and favors the growth of wanted bacteria, such a media is called enrichment media.

For example, tetrathionate broth, selenite F broth. These media inhibits coliforms (e.g. *Escherichia coli*) by allowing growth of pathogenic cultures from feces.

6. Selective media

They are like enrichment media but it is in solid form. When a substance is added to a solid medium which inhibits the growth of unwanted bacteria but permits the growth of required bacteria in the form of colonies is known as selective medium. Physical conditions of a culture media may be adjusted and made selective for the growth of specific micro-organisms, e.g. MacConkey's media (*Escherichia coli*).

7. Indicator Media

They contain an indicator which changes colour when a bacterial species grows in them, e.g. Wilson and Blair medium for *Salmonella typhi*, which reduces sulphite to sulphide in the presence of glucose and the colonies, have a black metallic shine.

8. Differential Media

It is used to distinguish between different types of bacteria based on some observable characteristics, e.g. MacConkey's medium. It shows lactose fermenter as red colonies while non lactose fermenter as white or pale colonies. Blood agar medium is an enriched medium but bacteria lysing red cells show a clearing around their colonies. Thus, it is an indicator medium or differential medium.

9. Transport Media

There are delicate microorganisms (e.g. *Neisseria gonorrhoeae*) which may not survive the time taken for transporting the specimen to the laboratory or may be overgrown by nonpathogens (*Escherichia coli*) and pathogens (*Salmonella species*).

Special media are devised for such type of delicate micro-organisms which are called transport media, e.g. Stuart's transport medium. Amies transport medium.

10. Assay Media

These media have specific compositions and are used for the assay of antibiotics, amino acids and vitamins. Media containing specific components are also used for testing disinfectants.

11. Storage Media

These media help in preservation and storage of bacteria for log period, e.g. Dorset's egg medium. Nutrient agar stabs, etc.

C. Physical Condition Required for the Nutrition and Growth

i. Gaseous Requirement

1. **Aerobic bacteria:** They require oxygen for growth and can grow when they are incubated in an air atmosphere (i.e. 2.1% oxygen).

2. **Anaerobic bacteria:** They do not use oxygen to obtain energy; moreover, oxygen is toxic for them. They cannot grow when incubated in an air atmosphere. *Non-stringent/ tolerant anaerobes:* They are those that tolerate low levels of oxygen.

   Stringent/strict anaerobes: They are those that cannot tolerate even low levels and may die upon brief exposure to air.

3. **Facultative anaerobic bacteria:** They do not require oxygen for growth; still they may use the oxygen for energy production if it is available. They are not inhibited by oxygen and usually grow well under an air atmosphere as like they grow in the absence of oxygen.

4. **Microaerophilic bacteria:** They require low levels of oxygen for growth but cannot tolerate the level of oxygen present in an air atmosphere.

ii. Temperature Requirement

1. **Psychrophiles:** They can grow at 0°C but have a optimum temperature 15°C or lower and maximum temperature of 20°C, e.g. *Vibrio psychroerythrus*.

   Psychrotrophic (facultative phsychrophile): These organisms are able to grow at 0°C but which grow best at temperature in the range of about 20–30°C, e.g. *Pseudomonas fluorescens*.

2. **Mesophiles:** These organisms can grow best within a temperature range of approximately 25–40°C. Most bacteria are growing best at about body temperature (37°C), e.g. *Corynebacterium diphtheriae*.

3. **Thermophiles:** They grow best at temperature above 45°C.

   Facultative thermophiles: The growth range of many thermophilic bacteria extends to the mesophilic region.

These species are called facultative thermophiles, e.g. *Streptococcus thermophilus*.

True/obligate/steno thermophiles: The thermophilic bacteria which cannot grow in mesophilic range are termed as true/obligate/steno thermophiles, e.g. *Thermus aquaticus.*

iii. pH Requirement

The pH of the growth medium of bacteria has a profound effect upon the multiplication of microorganisms. Each microbial species has definite pH range for growth and multiplication. Depending upon the optimum pH value of microorganisms, they can be classified as follows:

1. **Acidophiles:** These microorganisms have an optimum pH range in between 1 to 6.5, e.g. *Acidithiobacillus thiooxidans* (*Thiobacillus thiooxidans*) (pH 2–3.5).

2. **Neutrophils:** Most bacteria grow best in a narrow pH range between 6.5 and 7.5. Such bacteria are called neutrophils, e.g. *Escherichia coli, Salmonella typhi*, all pathogenic bacteria.

3. **Alkaliphiles:** These microorganisms have an optimum pH range in between 7.5 and 14, e.g. *Vibrio cholerae* (pH 9).

iv. Osmotic Pressure

Bacteria are more tolerant to osmotic variations because of the mechanical strength of the cell wall. They can grow in media with widely varying contents of salt, sugar and other solutes. Sudden exposure of bacteria to solutions of high salt concentrations may cause plasmolysis. Hence, 0.5% NaCl is added to almost all culture media to make the environment isotonic.

v. Light

Darkness is usually favorable for the growth and viability of all microorganisms. They are sensitive to ultraviolet radiation, direct light and other radiations.

XII. CULTIVATION OF BACTERIA

Cultivation of Autotrophs

The autotrophic bacteria exhibit the simplest requirements in terms of chemical as a nutritive substance for their growth. For example, the medium of the composition supports the growth of *Nitrosomonas europaea*. (This medium is called as chemically defined or synthetic medium because it is composed of known chemical compounds.) An organism can grow and reproduce in such a mixture of inorganic compounds indicates that it has an elaborate capacity for synthesis. For this, the organism can transform these compounds in to carbohydrate, proteins, nucleic acids, lipids, vitamins and other complex organic substances that constitute the living cells.

Cultivation of Heterotrophs

Although the heterotrophic bacteria constitute one major nutritional group, they vary considerably in the specific nutrients required for growth, particularly with respect to their organic carbon sources, nitrogen sources and vitamin requirements (Table 2.5).

Table 2.5: Cultivation of heterotrophs

Nutritional requirements	Species			
	E. coli	S. typhi	S. aureus	Lactobacillus
Inorganic salts	+	+	+	+
Organic carbon	+	+	+	+
Atmospheric nitrogen				
Inorganic nitrogen	+	+	+	+
One amino acid	+	+		
Two or more amino acids			+	+
One vitamin			+	
Two or more vitamins				+

The requirements may be relatively simple or complex, depending on the species (Table 2.5). For example, *E. coli* has much simpler nutritional requirements than *Lactobacilli*. Organism such as *Lactobacilli* that have elaborate requirements for specific nutrients, i.e. vitamins and other growth-promoting substances, are designated fastidious heterotrophs.

Cultivation of Aerobic Bacteria

To grow aerobic or facultative bacteria in tubes or small flasks, incubation of the medium under normal atmospheric conditions is generally satisfactory. However, when aerobic organisms are to be grown in large quantities, it is advantageous to increase the exposure of the medium to the atmosphere. This can be accomplished by dispensing the medium in shallow layers, for which special containers are available. Aeration can also be increased by constantly shaking the inoculated liquid cultures (Fig. 2.28).

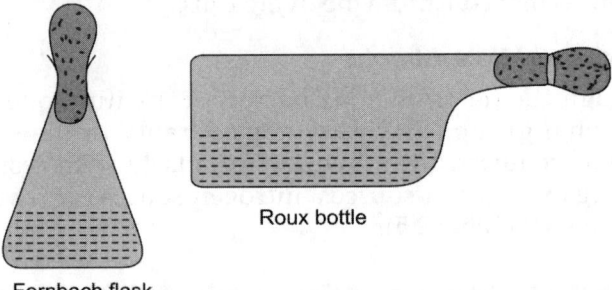

Roux bottle

Fernbach flask

Fig. 2.28: Cultivation of aerobic bacteria by providing a large surface area for a shallow layer of medium in culture vessels of several designs

Cultivation of Anaerobic Bacteria

Stringent anaerobes can be grown only by taking special precautions to exclude all atmospheric oxygen from the medium. Such environmental condition can be established by using one of the following methods:

1. **Prereduced media:** During preparation, the culture medium is boiled for several minutes to drive off most of the dissolved oxygen. A reducing agent, e.g. cysteine is added to further lower the oxygen content (Fig. 2.29).

   Oxygen free nitrogen is bubbled through the medium to keep it anaerobic. The medium is then dispensed into tubes which are being flushed with oxygen free nitrogen, stopper tightly and sterilized by autoclaving. Such tubes can be stored for many months before being used. During inoculation, the tubes are continuously flushed with oxygen free carbon dioxide by means or a cannula, restoppered, and incubated.

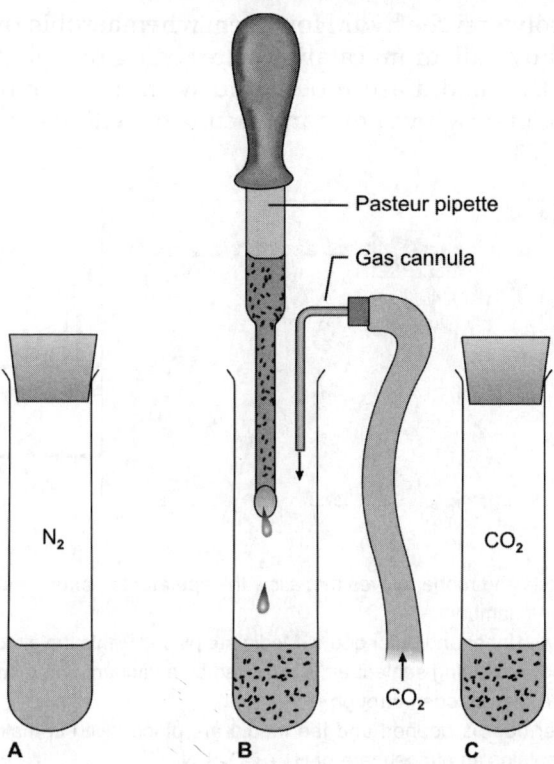

A. Tube of Prereduced medium containing an atmosphere of oxygen free nitrogen.

B. To inoculate, the stopper is removed and a gas cannula is inserted to flush the tube continuously with oxygen free carbon dioxide and maintain anaerobic condition. The medium is inoculated with a few drops of culture by means of a Pasteur pipette.

C. After inoculation the tube is re-stoppered and incubated.

Fig. 2.29: Cultivation of stringent anaerobes

2. **Anaerobic chamber:** This refers to a plastic anaerobic glove box that contains an atmosphere of hydrogen, carbon dioxide and nitrogen. Culture media are placed within the chamber by means of an air lock which can be evacuated and refilled with nitrogen.

From the air lock the media are placed within the main chamber. Any oxygen in the media is slowly removed by reaction with the hydrogen, forming water; this reaction is aided by palladium catalyst. After being rendered oxygen free, the media are inoculated within the chamber by means of the glove ports and incubated within the chamber (Fig. 2.30).

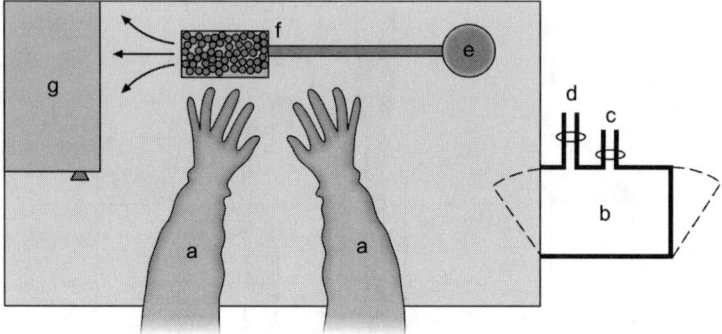

a. Glove ports and rubber gloves that allow the operator to perform manipulations within the chamber.
b. Air lock with inner and outer doors. Media are placed within the air lock with the inner door remaining sealed; air is removed by a vacuum pump connection
c. Replaced with nitrogen through
d. The inner door is opened and the media are placed with in main chamber, which contains an atmosphere of $H_2 + CO_2 + N_2$
e. A circulator that circulates the gas atmosphere through pellets of palladium catalyst
f. Causing any residual oxygen in the media to be used up by reaction with H_2.
g. Located within the chamber

Fig. 2.30: Anaerobic glove box

3. **Anaerobic jar:** Non-stringent anaerobes can be cultured within an anaerobic jar such as shown in Fig. 2.31.

   The inoculated media are placed in the jar along with a hydrogen and carbon dioxide generating system. After the jar is sealed, the oxygen present in the atmosphere within the jar, as well as that dissolved in the culture medium, is gradually used up through reaction with the hydrogen in the presence of a catalyst.

4. **Pyrogallate tubes and jars:** The two test tubes are joined in between by a joint. In one tube culture is placed and in other mixture of pyrogallic acid and sodium hydroxide is

placed. This mixture will ultimately scavenger oxygen from the internal environment and thus helps to generate the anaerobic condition.

Similar to the pyrogallate tubes, in pyrogallate jars the desiccator is used and the lower bottom is filled with mixture of pyrogallic acid and sodium hydroxide.

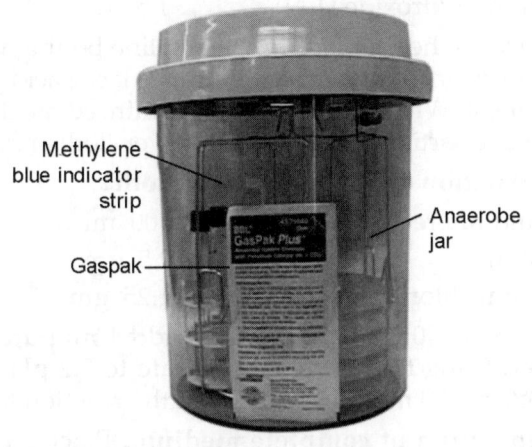

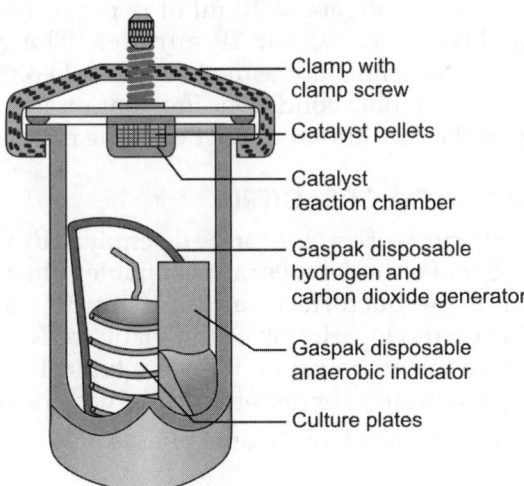

Fig. 2.31: Anaerobic jar

5. **Cooked meat medium (Robertson Bullock Heart Medium—RBHM):** It is a suitable medium for growing anaerobes and also for the preservation of stock of anaerobic micro-organisms.

a. **Preparation of cooked meat**

Fresh bovine heart	500 gms
Water	500 ml
Sodium hydroxide (1 N)	1.5 ml

Mince the heart, place in the alkaline boiling water and simmer for 20 minutes to neutralize lactic acid present in the meat. While still hot press the minced meat in a cloth and dry partially by spreading it over cloth or filter paper.

b. **Preparation of pepto infusion broth**

Liquid filtered from meat	500 ml
Peptone	2.5 gm
Sodium chloride	1.25 gm

Steam at 100 C for 20 minutes, add 1 ml pure HCl and filter. Bring the reaction of filtrate to 8.2 pH. Steam at 100°C for 30 minutes and adjust the reaction to pH 7.8.

c. **Preparation of complete medium:** Place meat in one ounce narrow neck bottle to level of about one inch and cover it with about 10 ml of pepto infusion broth. Autoclave at 121°C for 20 minutes. The oxidation reduction potential of the medium is –0.2 volts and thus it gives anaerobic condition. Inoculation is introduced deep in the medium in contact with the meat.

XIII. GROWTH CYCLE OF BACTERIA

Normal growth curve of bacteria can be determined by inoculating a small number of bacterial cells into a suitable culture medium and counting the bacteria in aliquot samples at regular intervals. When the logarithms of the viable cells are plotted against time on the graph paper, it gives a typical curve called as bacterial growth curve or growth cycle of bacteria (Fig. 2.32).

The resulting curve has four distinct phases

1. Lag phase
2. Log or logarithmic or exponential phase

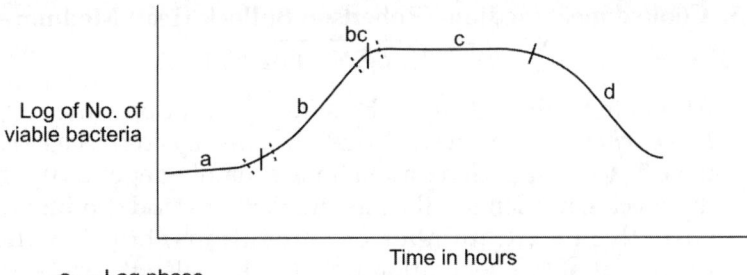

a — Lag phase
b — Log phase
c — Stationary phase
d — Death phase
bc — Transitional period

Fig. 2.32: Growth curve of bacteria

3. Stationary phase
4. Decline or death phase

1. **Lag phase:** When the bacteria are inoculated into a fresh medium, the microbial population remains constant for an initial period. The period between the inoculation and the beginning of multiplication is known as the *Lag phase*. In this phase, bacterial cells adjust itself to adopt the new environment. The enzymes, coenzymes and other essential molecules are synthesized by the bacterial cell during this phase. The cells are metabolically and physiologically very active but do not divide. The length of the lag phase depends upon the nature of medium species of microorganisms and other various physical and chemical growth factors.

2. **Log phase (exponential phase):** During this phase the cells divide steadily at a constant rate and the log of the number of the cells plotted against time results in a straight line. The bacteria multiply at their maximum rate and their number increases exponentially or by geometric progression with time. The time required for one bacterial division during this phase is known as generation time. The number of bacteria present in each generation period is almost twice that in the previous period.

The generation time (g) can be determined from the number of generations (n) that occur in a particular time (t).

$$g = \frac{t}{n} = \frac{t}{3.3\left(\text{Log } N - \text{Log } N_0\right)}$$

All bacteria do not have the same generation time, e.g. *Escherichia coli* may have 15–20 min, *Staphylococcus aureus* have 25 to 30 min. Generation time is mainly depends upon the species, nutrients in the medium and physical conditions. Growth rate (R, number of generations/hour) is the reciprocal of the generation time (g). It is also the slope of the straight line obtained when the Log number of cells plotted against time.

$$R = \frac{1}{g} = \frac{3.3\,\text{Log } N - \text{Log } N_0}{t}$$

3. **Stationary phase:** In this phase a constant high population of cells is maintained by the balance between the cell division and cell death. The rate of multiplication is reduced because depletion of nutrients, accumulation of toxic waste products, very high concentration of cells and low partial pressure of oxygen. A viable population count at this stage shows no change.

4. **Decline or death phase:** The death or decline phase is also known as the logarithmic death phase. During death phase, the number of viable cells decreases exponentially, essentially the inverse of growth during the Log phase. A variety of conditions contribute to the bacterial death but the most important are depletion of nutrients and accumulation of toxic waste products. Bacteria die at different rates, just as they grow at the different rates.

   Between each of these phases, there is a small curved portion called the transitional period.

Types of growth

There are mainly three types of growth:
1. Synchronous growth
2. Diauxic growth
3. Continuous growth

1. **Synchronous growth:** The synchronous growth is the growing of microorganisms in such a way that they are all

in same stage of growth phase and all will divide at same time with respect to each other. Thus, the entire population is kept uniform with respect to growth and division. It is not possible to analyze a single bacterial cell to obtain the information about the growth behavior, i.e. organization, differentiation and macromolecular synthesis. Synchronous culture provides the entire cell crop in the same stage of growth. Fig. 2.33 shows the growth pattern of the population of synchronous cells. The synchrony is generally lost after a few generations.

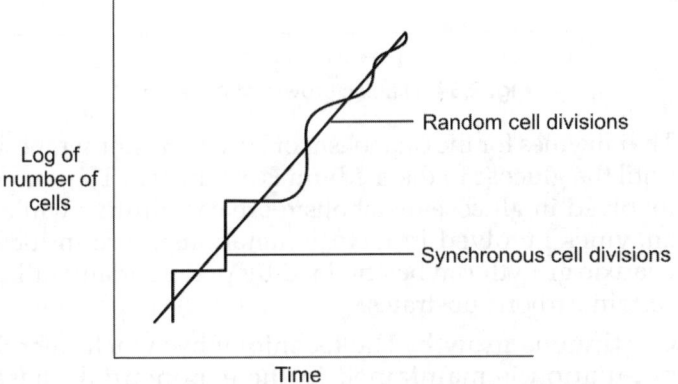

Fig. 2.33: Synchronous growth of bacteria

Measurements made on such cultures are equivalent to the measurements made on individual cells. Synchronous population can be generated either by physically separating cells in the same stage of division or by forcing a cell population to attain an identical, physiological condition by a change in the environment. Physical separation of the cells by centrifugation, filtration or by periodic changes in nutritional and environmental conditions produces synchronously dividing cell populations.

2. **Diauxic growth:** Bacterial growth characterized by two separate phases due to the preferential use of one carbon source over another is called as diauxic growth. In 1942, *Jacques Monod* discovered the phenomenon of "diauxy".

In a medium containing glucose and lactose, microbes first uses glucose and lactose is not the metabolized until all the glucose is used up (Fig. 2.34).

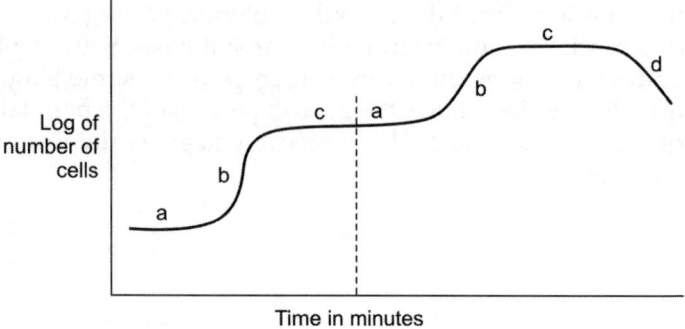

Fig. 2.34: Diauxic growth of bacteria

The enzymes for the catabolism of lactose are not synthesized until the glucose in the medium is exhausted. The enzymes involved in glucose metabolism are constitutive while the enzymes involved in lactose metabolism are inducible. Diauxic growth can be obtained by preferentially utilizing certain carbon substrates.

3. **Continuous growth:** The technique by which microbial population is maintained in the exponential phase of growth in a constant environment is known as continuous culture technique. It is necessary to maintain a bacterial population in the exponential or Log phase for research and industry processes. This condition is known as steady state growth.

XV. REPRODUCTION OF BACTERIA

Bacteria reproduce asexually as well as sexually. A bacterial reproduction takes place by the following methods:
1. Binary fission
2. Budding
3. Fragmentation
4. Formation of conidiospores or sporangiospores

1. **Binary fission:** Microorganism multiplies by the asexual process of cell fission which results in division of the cell

into two or more vegetative cells. Most bacteria multiply by transverse binary fission that is division into two equal cells. The circular chromosome divides into two identical circles, which segregate at apposated ends of the cell (Fig. 2.35).

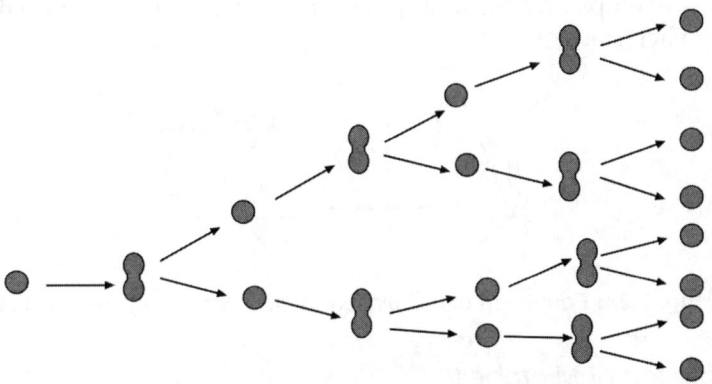

Fig. 2.35: Multiplication by binary fission

Simultaneously, the cell wall is laid down in the middle of the cell, which finally grows to produce two new cells each with its own wall and nucleus, e.g. *Bacillus subtilis, Enterococcus faecalis.*

2. **Budding:** It is a process in which a small bud develops at one end of the cell is called budding (Fig. 2.36). This bud enlarges and eventually develops into a new cell which separates from the parent, e.g. Baker's yeast (*Saccharomyces cerevisiae*), *Rhodopseudomonas acidophila, Hyphomicrobium vulgare.*

3. **Fragmentation:** Bacteria may produce extensive filamentous growth and reproduce by fragmentation of the filaments into small bacillary or coccoid cells (Fig. 2.37). Each filament grows and forms a new cells, e.g. *Nocardia* species.

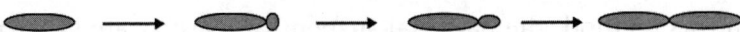

Fig. 2.36: Budding of bacteria

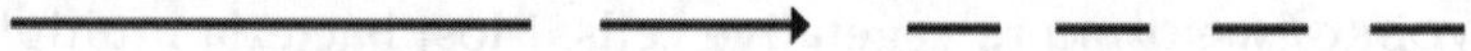

Fig. 2.37: Reproduction by fragmentation

4. **Formation of conidiospores or sporangiospores:** Some
   bacteria produce may spores per organism by developing
   cross walls at the hyphal tips (Fig. 2.38). Each spore
   develops and form new cells, e.g. *Streptomyces* and related
   bacteria.

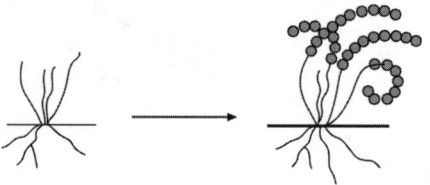

Fig. 2.38: Formation of conidiospores by a *Streptomyces* species

Isolation of Microbes

Isolation refers to the separation of specific microorganism
from heterogeneous population. Microorganisms are generally
found in nature in mixed population. So for detail study, it
is important to separate the particular microorganism
species. Methods of isolation are different for each group of
microbes.

XVI. ISOLATION OF BACTERIA

The methods widely used for the isolation of bacteria are as
follows:
1. Streak plate method
2. Pour plate method
3. Spread plate method
4. Roll tube method
5. Heating culture at 70°C
6. Cultivation on differential media

1. Streak Plate Method

In this method, the bacterial suspension is separated on the
solid media by inoculating the needle in various ways.

Types of streaking

- Simple streaking
- Streaking in quadrants
- Streaking in grids

Methodology

Sterilize the wire loop by holding it in Bunsen burner flame and cool for a few second. Aseptically remove a loopful of culture with wire loop. Raise the lid of sterile nutrient agar containing plate just high enough to insert the wire loop. With free arm movement spread the culture at one corner of plate. Then draw the first streak in the first quadrant. Likewise, streak in draw 2nd, 3rd, and 4th quadrants. After each streak sterilize and cool the wire loop. The first streak will contain more number of microbes. The last streak should thin out the culture to give isolated colonies. Such inoculated nutrient agar petri plate is then allowed to incubate at proper temperature and time. On the last streak well-isolated colonies will appear. Each colony represents pure growth of organism.

2 . Pour Plate Method

Dilution of sample

The dilution of sample is important step for this method. Take 1 gm/ml of sample; aseptically mix it with 99 ml sterile saline. This leads to 1:100 dilution of sample. Add 1ml of this mixture into tube containing 9 ml sterile saline with the help of sterile pipette. This leads to 1:1000 dilutions. Make several dilutions as above (1:10000 to 1:1000000). Select any dilution for the further experiments (Fig. 2.39).

Methodology

Take 1ml mixture from any of dilution (e.g. 1:10000) with the help of sterile pipette. Inoculate it into sterile nutrient agar butt at 45°C (nutrient agar butt contains approximately 20 ml nutrient agar medium) in a tube, maintained in liquefied condition at 50°C. Shake the nutrient agar butt to distribute the sample properly. Pour the content in sterile empty Petri-plate and allow solidifying. Incubate the plate at proper temperature for 24 hours. Analyze the colonies qualitatively and quantitatively. Calculate the number of colonies on the agar surface. This will

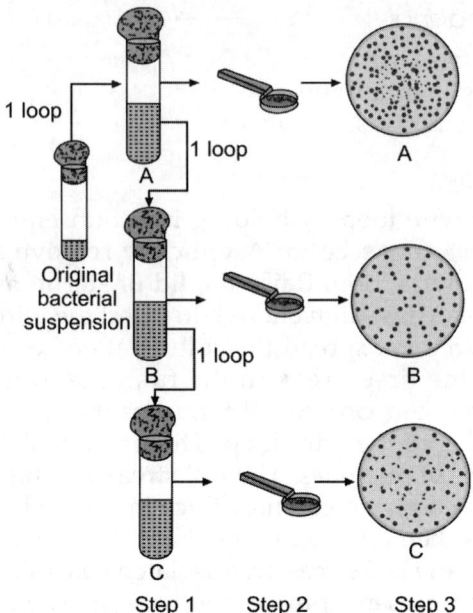

1 loop

1 loop

A

Original
bacterial
suspension

1 loop

B

C

Step 1   Step 2   Step 3

Fig. 2.39: Isolation of bacteria by streak plate method

give the number of microorganisms in diluted sample. To calculate the total number of microorganisms in the initial sample, multiply the number of colonies by diluting factor.

Disadvantages

1. The microorganisms are subjected to hot shock because liquid medium is maintained at 45°C temperature.
2. This method is unsuitable for isolating psychrophile type of bacteria.
3. This method is tedious, time consuming and requires skilled hands.
4. The microorganisms are trapped beneath the surface of the medium when it solidifies. So, the surface and subsurface colonies are developed and it is very difficult to isolate and count the subsurface colonies.

3. Spread Plate Method

In this technique, the bacterial suspension is uniformly distributed on solid agar by glass spreader (Fig. 2.40).

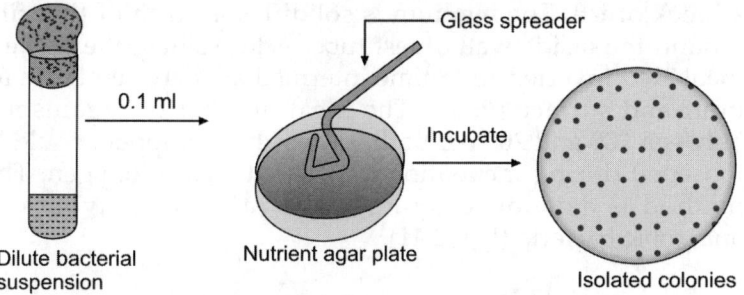

Fig. 2.40: Isolation of bacteria by spread plate technique

Methodology

With the help of a sterile pipette, add 1 ml of given sample into sterile 99 ml saline containing flask and then add 1ml of this mixture into 9ml saline containing tubes. Repeat the process for several times to achieve a specific dilution. Place 0.1ml of any prepared dilution on sterile nutrient agar plate with the help of a sterile pipette. Sterilize a glass spreader by flaming and allow it to cool between two burners. Then spread the drop of suspension uniformly over the agar surface with the help of sterilized spreader. Incubate the petri plate for 24 hours at appropriate temperature and observe it on next day. Calculate the number of colonies on agar surface. This will give the number of microorganisms in diluted sample. To calculate the total number of microorganisms in the initial sample, multiply the number of colonies by dilution factor.

Advantages

1. For many purposes a bacterial lawn-dense bacterial growth is required (e.g. in microbiological assay). This method is appropriate for this purpose.
2. Only surface colonies are developed and hence easy to pick them up.
3. It is possible to enumerate the number of microorganisms in any given suspension by this method.

4. Roll Tube Method

Roll tubes are prepared by adding the dilution of organisms to a small volume of nutrient agar in a test tube, shaking to mix the contents and rotating horizontally, under cold water or in a block of ice. The medium is solidifies in form of thin film around the inside wall of test tube. After rolling, the bottle is incubated inverted for a time intermediate between those for pour and surface plates. The ideal number of organism is between 100 and 200 per bottle. The rubber stopper should be loosened during incubation to prevent lack of oxygen. This method is developed by *R. E. Hungate* for cultivation of anaerobic bacteria (Fig. 2.41).

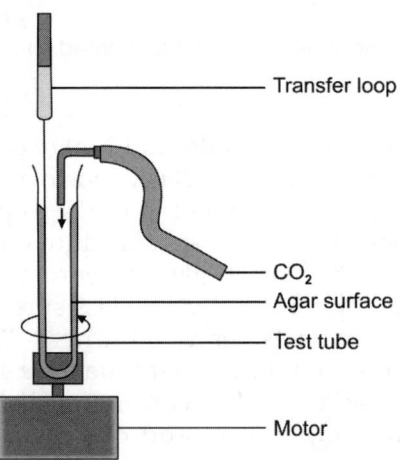

Fig. 2.41: Isolation of bacteria by roll tube method

Methodology

Take test tube containing a few milliliters of molten agar medium. The medium should be reduced chemically to remove dissolved oxygen. This is possible by incorporation of several chemicals like sodium thioglycollate. The tube is tightly closed with butyl rubber bung (to maintain anaerobic condition). The molten agar is inoculated with appropriate dilution of source of bacteria by inserting them through the rubber stopper with sterile syringe. The tubes are then laid on their sides in ice and rolled until the agar solidifies in thin layer on the wall of tube. This procedure leads to separation of the microbes. After incubation when colonies become visible, the bung is removed and isolated colonies are picked from agar with a needle or capillary tube. Whenever a tube is opened, entry of air is prevented by continuous passing stream of CO_2

or N_2 into tube. To ensure anaerobic condition, dye-like resazurin must be incorporated into medium.

Advantages

1. Many bacteria are killed by even momentary exposure of air. Cultivation of such microbes in routine atmospheric condition and by general technique is not possible.
2. It is the widely used method for isolation of anaerobes.

5. Heating Culture at 70°C

The non spore forming bacteria will be killed and only the spore forming bacteria which can resist the temperature will survive.

6. Cultivation on Differential Media

Selective medium will enhance the growth of one type of microbes and suppresses the growth of other type of microbes.

Example: On Penicillin agar media only the gram-negative bacteria can grow as gram-positive bacteria will be destroyed by antibiotic.

Selective media	Microbe which can grow
Blood tellurite agar	C. diphtheriae
Deoxycitrate medium	Salmonella and Shigella
Bismuth sulphite agar	Salmonella typhi
Lowenstein Jensen medium	M. tuberculosis
Dorset egg medium	M. tuberculosis

Differential media are the medium that distinguish between groups of bacteria and even permits their identification, e.g. MacConkey's agar.

XVII. VIRUSES

The word virus is derived from a Latin root meaning a slimy, noxious liquid, sort of living snake venom. Viruses cause man diseases of humans, animals and plants. They are unique group of infectious agent. They are not cellular pathogens or parasites of bacteria, animals and plants. A complete virus particle or a virion consists of one or more molecules of DNA or RNA in a coat protein Virus can exist in two phases

1. Extracellular
2. Intracellular

In extracellular phase, virus may not possess enzyme. If it contains, it may be a few enzymes, virus cannot reproduce independently of living cells. In an intracellular phase, the viral nucleic acid replicates. Then it induces first all metabolisms to synthesize the various viral components. All the components are assembled to produce a complete virion or a virus particle. Then they release out of living microorganism.

A. General Characteristics of Viruses

1. Viruses contain a single type of nucleic acid, either DNA or RNA, never both.
2. They contain a protein coat.
3. They multiply inside living cells using the synthesizing machinery of the cell.
4. They cause the synthesis of specialized structures that can transfer the viral nucleic acid to other cells.
5. They are easily transmitted from one organism to another, and they are not affected by antibiotics
6. They reproduce solely through their nucleic acid and are unable to grow or undergo binary fission.

B. Classification of Virus

i. Depending upon their Primary Characteristics

1. **Depending upon the chemical nature of nucleic acid,** e.g. RNA or DNA, single or double stranded, single or segmented genome, (+) or (−) strand, molecular weight. Table 2.6 describes characteristic of different viruses.
2. **Depending upon the structure of virus:** Virus may be classified into different types, depending on the capsid structure
   a. *Helical viruses:* Helical viruses resemble long rods that may be rigid or flexible. The viral nucleic acid is found within a hollow, cylindrical capsid, which has a helical structure (Fig. 2.42), e.g. *Rabies virus, Tobacco mosaic virus.*
   b. *Polyhedral (icosahedral virus):* The capsids of most polyhedral viruses have a shape of an icosahedron, a regular polyhedron with 20 triangular faces and 12 corners (Fig. 2.43). The capsomers of each face form an equilateral triangle, e.g. *Adenovirus, Poliovirus.*

Table 2.6: Characteristic of viruses

Class	Nucleic acid	Shape	Example
1. RNA viruses			
I(a)	(+), ss RNA	Icosahedral	*Picornavirus*
I(b)	(+), ss RNA	Icosahedral	*Togaviruses*
II	(−), ss RNA	Helical	*Paramyxovirus*
III	(−), ss RNA	Helical	*Orthomyxovirus*
IV			
2. DNA virus	ds, RNA*	Icosahedral	*Reovirus*
I(a)	ds, linear DNA	Icosahedral	*Adenovirus*
I(b)	ds, linear DNA	Icosahedral	*Herpesvirus*
I(c)	ds, linear DNA	Complex	*Poxvirus*
II	ds, circular DNA	Icosahedral	*Papovavirus*
III	ss, linear DNA	Icosahedral	*Parvovirus*

* Segmented, ds: double stranded, ss: single stranded

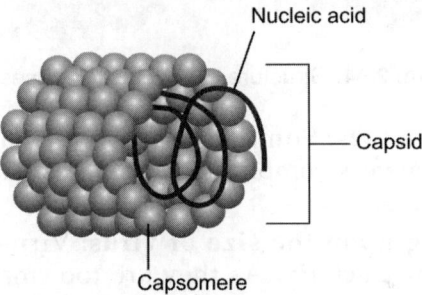

Fig. 2.42: Structure of helical viruses

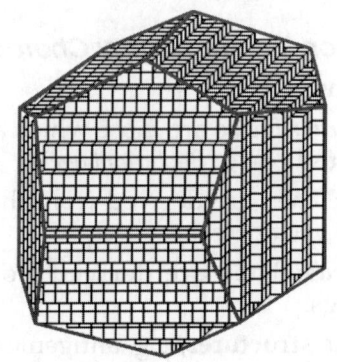

Fig. 2.43: Structure of polyhedral viruses

c. Enveloped viruses: They are roughly spherical but highly pleomorphic (variable in shape) in nature. When helical or polyhedral viruses are enclosed by envelopes, they are called enveloped helical (e.g. *Influenza virus*) and enveloped polyhedral viruses (e.g. *Herpes simplex virus*) (Fig. 2.44).

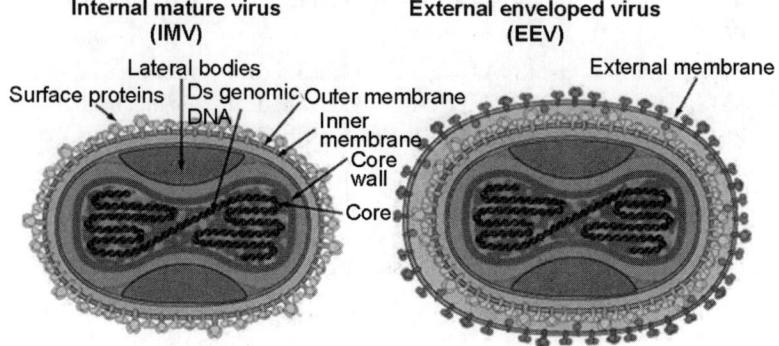

Fig. 2.44: Structure of enveloped viruses

d. Complex viruses: Some viruses, particularly bacterial viruses have very complicated structures. They are called complex virus.

3. **Depending upon the size of virus:** Viruses are much smaller than bacteria. As they are too small to be seen under the light microscope, they are called *ultramicroscopic* (Fig. 2.45).

ii. Depending upon the Secondary Characteristic of Virus

1. **Host range:** Host specific

a. *Bacterial virus:* These are those which are derived from the host bacteria, (e.g. *Bacteriophage*)

b. *Plant virus:* They are derived from the host plant cell (e.g. *Tobacco mosaic virus*)

c. *Animal Virus:* They are derived from the animals, human beings.

2. **Specific surface structures,** e.g. antigenic properties

3. **Mode of transmission,** e.g. feces

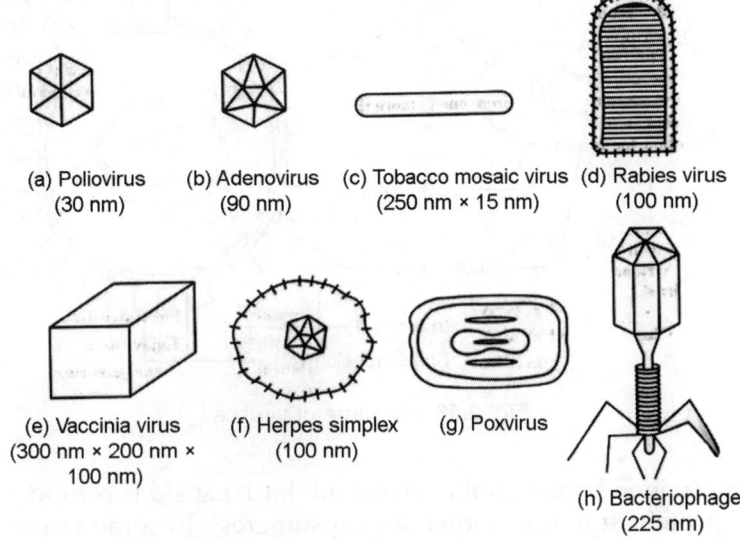

(a) Poliovirus
(30 nm)

(b) Adenovirus
(90 nm)

(c) Tobacco mosaic virus
(250 nm × 15 nm)

(d) Rabies virus
(100 nm)

(e) Vaccinia virus
(300 nm × 200 nm × 100 nm)

(f) Herpes simplex
(100 nm)

(g) Poxvirus

(h) Bacteriophage
(225 nm)

Fig. 2.45: Classification of viruses depending upon size of virus

XVIII. STRUCTURE OF VIRUSES

A virion is the complete, fully developed viral particle composed of nucleic acid surrounded by a coat that protects it from the environment and serves as a vehicle of transmission from one host cell to another host cell. Virus are not cellular and therefore do not have a nucleus, cytoplasm or cell membrane (Fig. 2.46).

Nucleic acid

Virus contains a single kind of nucleic acid, either DNA or RNA, which is the genetic material.

The percentage of nucleic acid in relation to protein is about 1% of the influenza viruses and about 50% of certain Bacteriophages. The nucleic acid of a virus can be single stranded or double stranded. Depending on the viruses, the nucleic acid can be linear or circular. In some viruses (e.g. *influenza*), the nucleic acid is in separate segments

Capsid and envelope

The nucleic acid of viruses is surrounded by a protein coat which is called 'capsid'. The structure of capsid is ultimately

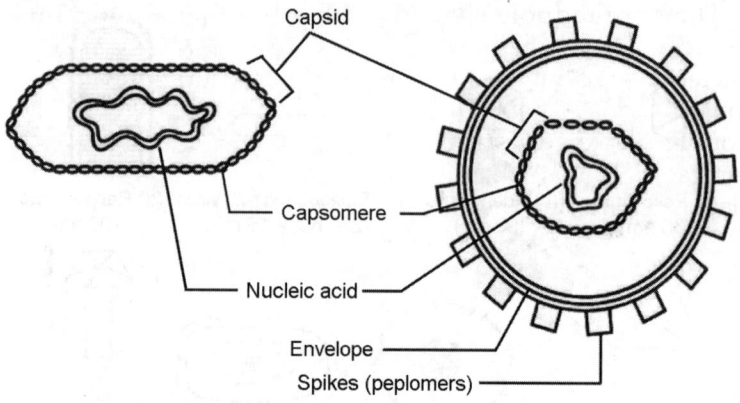

Fig. 2.46: Structure of viruses

determined by the viral nucleic acid. Each capsid is composed of protein subunits known as 'capsomeres'. In some viruses, the proteins composing the capsomeres are of a single type, in other viruses, many types of proteins may be present. In some viruses, the capsid is covered by an envelope, which usually consists of some combination of lipids, proteins and carbohydrates. Some animal viruses are released from the host cell and coats the virus with a layer of the host cells plasma membrane, that layer becomes the viral envelope.

Depending upon the virus, envelopes may or may not be covered by spikes. Spikes are carbohydrate protein complexes that project from the surface of the enveloped. Some virus attach to the host cell by means of spikes. The viruses whose capsids are not covered by an envelope are known as 'necked viruses' or non-enveloped viruses'.

XIX. BACTERIOPHAGE

Bacteriophage viruses are those which infect bacteria. Bacteriophage like all viruses composed of a nucleic acid surrounded by a protein coat. Bacteriophage are bacterial viruses occur in different shapes, although many have a tail through which they inoculate the host cell with viral nucleic acid. Bacteriophage is having very complicated structure. These are called *complex viruses*.

They are tadpole shaped, with a hexagonal head and a cylindrical tail. The head consists of a tightly packed core of nucleic acid (double stranded DNA) surrounded by a protein coat or capsid. The size of the head varies in different phages from 28 nm to 100 nm. The tail composed of a hollow core, a contractile sheath surrounding the core and a terminal base plate which has attached to it prongs, tail fibers or both (Fig. 2.47).

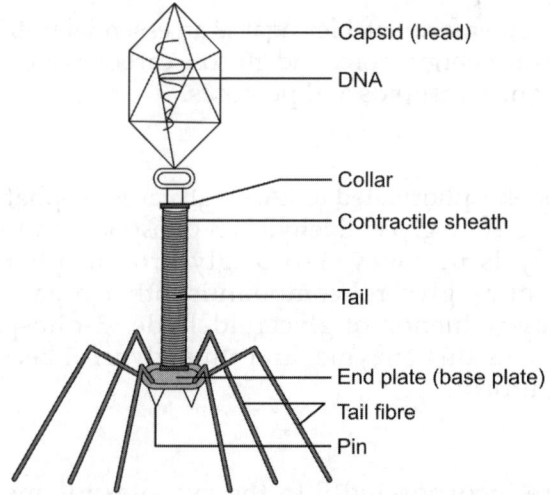

Fig. 2.47: Structure of T-even bacteriophage viruses

Bacteriophages are of two types:
1. Lytic or virulent
2. Temperate or avirulent

1. **Lytic or virulent:** This bacteriophage when infect the bacterial cell, large number of new viruses are produced inside the bacterial cell. At the end of incubation period, host cell bursts or lyses and releases new bacteriophage. These new bacteriophage will infect the other host cell. This is called Lytic cycle.

2. **Temperate or avirulent or lysogenic:** The viral nucleic acid is carried and replicated in the host bacterial cell. The transmitted from one generation to another without any cell lysis.

XX. NUTRITIONAL REQUIREMENT OF VIRUS

The medium used in the preparation of viral pool is of the following composition:

1. Enzymatic lactalbumin hydrolysate, 0.25%
2. Yeastolate, 0.05%; calf serum 5%
3. Eagle's basal serum 94.7%

Glucose

Glucose or other fermentable sugar is an essential nutrient. It is required as an energy source and glucose carbon is incorporated into galactan, glycolipids and pentoses.

Glycerol

Glycerol is phosphorylated to L-α-3- glycerophosphate, which is then oxidized to glyceraldehydes-3-phosphate and so enters the glycolysis pathway. L-α-3- glycerophosphate is the precursor of all glycerol compounds; other organisms can obtain it by reduction of glyceraldehydes-3-phospate, but *mycoides* lacks this enzyme, and thus glycerol becomes an essential nutrient.

Lipid

Sterols are incorporated into the cytoplasmic membrane without change in structure. Most of the bound fatty acids can be removed and pure fatty acids can be added to the medium together with defatted serum albumin to provide a non-toxic medium of known fatty acid composition. Therefore, it was sound that good growth could be obtained when certain pairs of fatty acids—a straight chain saturated fatty acid and the other *cis*-monoenoic fatty acid were supplied. Any single fatty acid or combination of fatty acids supports growth, provided that, at the growth temperature, the fluidity of membrane lipids lies within certain limits.

Nucleic acid precursor, vitamins and amino acids

The use of defatted serum albumin or other fatty acid binding proteins had a disadvantage of obscuring the requirement of amino acids. A completely defined medium was developed in which serum albumin and free fatty acids were replaced by a mixture of synthetic diacetoxysuccinyl esters of monoolein and monopalmitin. For vitamins and co-factors, thiamine, riboflavin and nicotinic acid were essential as a co-enzyme A. No requirement was found for folic acid or its derivatives.

XXI. CULTIVATION OF VIRUSES

Viruses are obligate intracellular parasites, which cannot be grown on inanimate culture media.

A. Cultivation of Animal Virus

Three methods are used for the cultivation of viruses.
1. Laboratory animals
2. Embryonated eggs
3. Tissue culture

1. **Laboratory animals:** Cultivation of viruses in living organism is the oldest method. Animals used for the cultivation of viruses are human volunteers usually for yellow fever virus, monkeys, mice, infant mice, rabbits, guinea pigs and ferrets. Use of these animals is not permitted due to the regulations of animal ethics committee.

   Animal inoculation is use for identifying and isolation from the clinical specimen. Animal are inoculated with specimens and growth of virus may be observed by sign of death, disease or visible lesions. Sometimes immunity in the experimental animal may interfere with the growth of viruses in the animal. Animal inoculation is also used for the study of pathogenesis, immune response and epidemiology.

2. **Embryonated eggs:** The embryonated egg offers several sites for the cultivation of viruses (Fig. 2.48).

   A hole is drilled in the shell of embryonated egg. Viral suspension is injected into the respective membrane or respective cavity of egg which is most appropriate for the growth of virus. Viral growth in embryonated egg is indicated by cell damage, death of embryo, or formation of typical pock marks/lesion on the egg membrane.

   This method is widely used for viral preparation and growth and also for some viral vaccines.

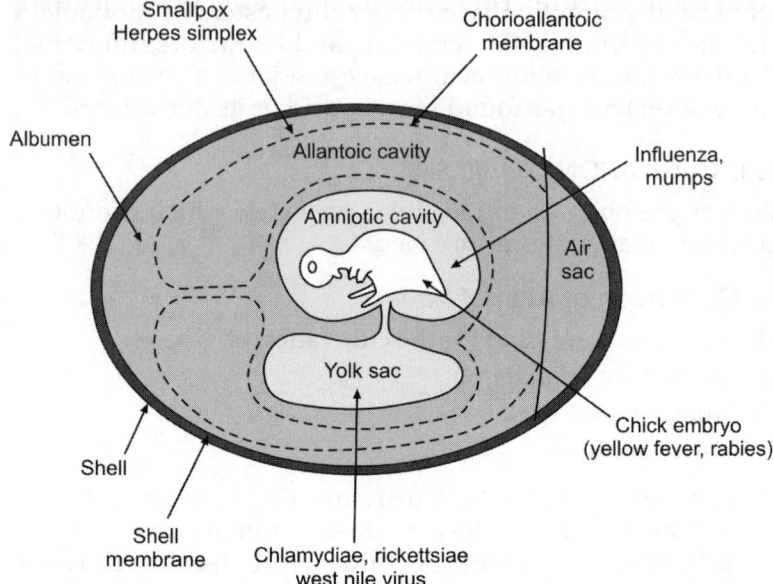

Fig. 2.48: A chick embryo showing the inoculation route for virus cultivation

Advantages of embryonated eggs

1. The eggs are much simpler to handle than animals.
2. Eggs are very economical and easily available.
3. They do not need feeding and caging.
4. They do not have an immune mechanism like animals to counteract virus infection.
5. They are clean and bacteriologically sterile.
6. Chick embryo offers several sites for cultivation of viruses.

Disadvantages of embryonated eggs

1. Some viruses do not show growth on primary inoculation into the eggs.
2. Slight amount of bacterial contamination in the inoculums may kill the embryo.
3. Eggs may be contaminated with mycoplasma and latent fowl viruses which may interfere with the growth of other viruses.

3. Tissue culture: There are mainly three types of tissue cultures:

1. Organ culture
2. Explants culture
3. Cell culture

1. *Organ culture:* Organ cultures are useful for the isolation of some viruses which appear to be highly specialized parasites of certain organs, e.g. tracheal ring organ culture is used for isolation of corona virus.

2. *Explants culture:* Minced tissue may be grown as explants embedded in plasma clots. This is not useful in virology. But in past, the adenoid tissue explants cultures were used for adenovirus.

3. *Cell culture:* This is a very popular and useful technique routinely used for cultivation of viruses. Tissues are dissociated into the component cells by the action of proteolytic enzymes such as trypsin and mechanical shaking. The cells are washed, counted and suspended in a growth medium and distributed in Petri plates, test tubes or bottles. The cells adhere to the glass surface and grow out to form a monolayer sheet.

Depending upon their origin and characteristics, cell cultures are classified into three types:

1. Primary cell cultures: These are normal cells freshly taken from the body and cultured. They are capable of only limited growth in a culture and cannot be maintained in serial culture (Fig. 2.49).

   They are useful for isolation and cultivation of viruses for vaccine production.

   For example, Rhesus monkey kidney cell culture, human embryonic kidney cell culture, human amnion cell, chick embryo fibroblast culture, etc.

2. Diploid cell strains: Diploid cell cultures are derived from primary cell cultures and established from a particular type of tissue, such as lung and kidney, which is embryonic in origin. The primary cell culture is transferred to the nutritive medium of cell culture and the process is called as sub-culturing. This cell culture, obtained

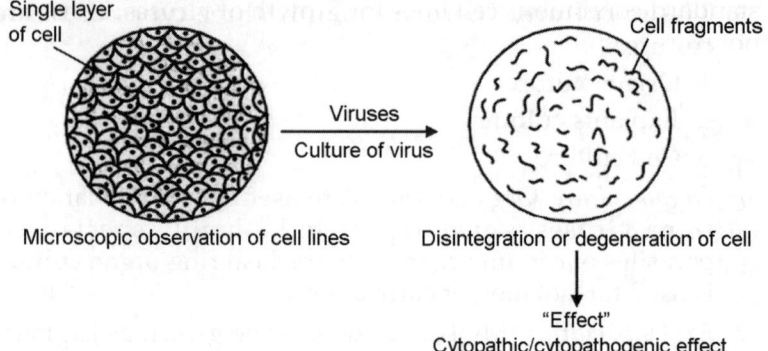

Single layer of cell

Cell fragments

Viruses
Culture of virus

Microscopic observation of cell lines

Disintegration or degeneration of cell

"Effect"
Cytopathic/cytopathogenic effect

Fig. 2.49: Cytopathic effect of a virus in a tissue culture cell

by sub-culturing of primary cell culture is called secondary cell.

Sub-culturing can be performed for 50 generations after which primary cells die out. They possess the normal diploid karyotype. They are useful for the isolation of fastidious pathogens and also for the production of viral vaccines.

For example, cell culture derived from human embryo is generally used for production of rabies vaccine. By sub-culturing, cells up to 100 generations can be made. They are used for culturing those viruses which require a human host.

3. Continuous cell lines: They are single type of cells mainly derived from cancer cells. These also can be grown in successive generations by transferring them from one test tube to another test tube without change in the character of cells. They have potential for unlimited growth and multiplication (Fig. 2.48).

These can be maintained indefinitely in a laboratory. The cell lines may be maintained by serial sub-cultivation in nutritive medium or stored in a cold for (–70°C), e.g. human carcinoma or cervix cell line (HeLa), baby hamster kidney cell line (BAK 21), human carcinoma of nasopharynx line (KB), human epithelioma of larynx cell line (Hep-2), etc.

All these cell lines are maintained in the labs all ones the world for the cultivation of viruses. These are considered as standard continuous cell lines for growth of viruses. These are not used for preparation of viral vaccines as vaccines prepared in cancer cells are considered unsafe for human use.

B. Cultivation of Bacteriophages (Bacterial Virus)

These are cultivated in either broth or agar cultures of young actively growing bacterial cell. Agar cultures are prepared by mixing the bacteriophage sample with cool, liquid agar and a suitable bacterial culture. The mixture is quickly poured into a petridish containing bottom layer of sterile agar.

After hardening, a bacterium in the top layer of agar grows and reproduces, forming a continuous, opaque layer or lawn. Whenever a virus comes to rest in the top agar, the viruses infects a bacterial cell and reproduce. Bacterial lysis will be resulted and this leads to the clearing in the lawn and plaques will form.

C. Cultivation of Plant Viruses

Plant viruses are cultivated in a variety of ways i.e., plant tissue cultures, cultures of separated cells or cultures of protoplasts may be used. Viruses can also be grown in wide plants, e.g. leaves are mechanically inoculated when rubbed with mixture of viruses and an abrasive such as carborundum. When all the walls are broken by the abrasion, the viruses directly contact the plasma membrane and infect the host cells. A localized necrotic lesion often develops due to rapid death of cells in the infected area. When lesions do not arise, the infected plant may show symptoms such as change in pigmentation or change in leaf shape.

XXII. MULTIPLICATION OF BACTERIAL VIRUS (BACTERIOPHAGE)/ LIFE CYCLE OF BACTERIOPHAGES

Bacteriophage exhibit two different types of life cycles (Fig. 2.50).

1. **Lytic or virulent cycle:** In this cycle, there is intracellular multiplication of phages followed by lysis and release of progeny virions. This is called 'lytic cycle' (Fig. 2.51).

2. **Lysogenic of avirulent or temperate cycle:** In this cycle the bacterial phage DNA becomes integrated with the bacterial genome, replicating synchronously without any cell lysis.

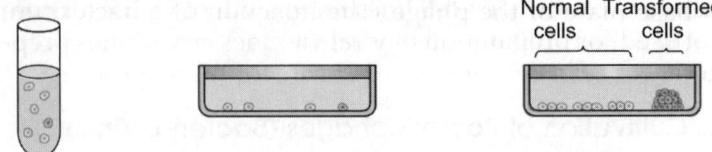

1 A tissue is treated with enzymes to separate the cells

2 Cells are suspended in culture medium

3 Normal cells or primary cells grow in a monolayer across the glass or plastic container. Transformed cells or continuous cell cultures do not grow in a monolayer

Fig. 2.50: Continuous cell lines

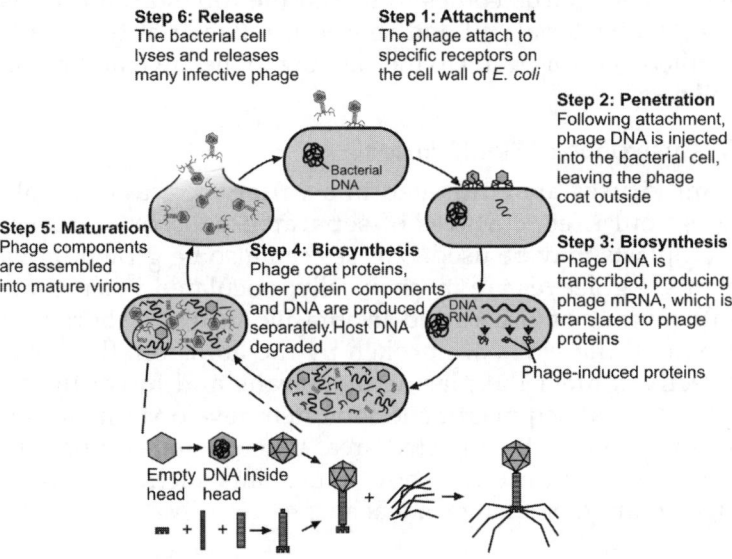

Step 6: Release
The bacterial cell lyses and releases many infective phage

Step 1: Attachment
The phage attach to specific receptors on the cell wall of *E. coli*

Step 2: Penetration
Following attachment, phage DNA is injected into the bacterial cell, leaving the phage coat outside

Step 5: Maturation
Phage components are assembled into mature virions

Step 4: Biosynthesis
Phage coat proteins, other protein components and DNA are produced separately. Host DNA degraded

Step 3: Biosynthesis
Phage DNA is transcribed, producing phage mRNA, which is translated to phage proteins

Fig. 2.51: Lytic growth cycle of bacteriophage

i. Lytic or Virulent Cycle/Multiplication of Bacteriophages

1. **Attachment or adsorption:** The first step in infections of a host bacterial cell by a bacteriophage is called as adsorption. *Bacteriophage* particles come into contact with bacterial cells by random collision. A phage attaches to the surface of a susceptible bacterium by its tail. Adsorption depends upon the presence of complementary chemical groups on the receptor sites of the bacterial surface and on the terminal

base plate of the phage. The infection of a bacterium by the naked phage nucleic acid is known as 'transfection' (Fig. 2.52).

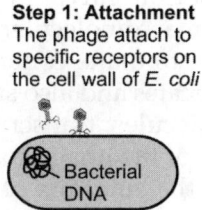

Step 1: Attachment
The phage attach to specific receptors on the cell wall of *E. coli*

Bacterial DNA

Fig. 2.52: Attachment and adsorption

2. **Penetration:** Attachment is followed by injection of DNA (Nucleic acid) into the bacterial cell. The phage DNA is injected into the bacterial body through the hollow core. Penetration may be facilitated by the presence of the bacteriophage tail of lysozyme which breaks a portion of the bacterial cell wall for the entry of the bacterial phage DNA. The phage DNA alone is necessary for the initiation of the synthesis of daughter phages (Fig. 2.53).

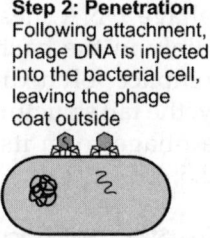

Step 2: Penetration
Following attachment, phage DNA is injected into the bacterial cell, leaving the phage coat outside

Fig. 2.53: Penetration

After penetration of DNA the empty head and tail of the bacteriophage remain outside the bacteria called 'shell or ghost'. If many bacteriophages are attached to the bacterial cell, multiple holes are produced on the cell with the consequent leakage of the cell contents. Bacterial lysis occurs without viral multiplication. This is known as 'lysis from without'. The bacteriophage such as T_1 and T_5, that do not have a contractile sheath also inject their nucleic acid through the cell envelope by adhesion sites between the inner and outer membrane.

3. **Biosynthesis of phage components:** After infection and penetration of DNA, transcription of a part of the viral genome produces 'early mRNA molecules, which are translated into a set of 'early' proteins. These serve to switch off host cell macromolecular synthesis, degrade the host DNA and start to make components for viral DAN. The viral DNA replicates and also starts to produce a batch of 'late' mRNA molecules, transcribed from genes which specify the proteins of the phage coat. These late messages are translated into the subunits of the capsid structures, which condense to form phage heads, tails and tail fibers (Fig. 2.54).

Step 3: Biosynthesis
Phage DNA is transcribed, producing phage mRNA, which is translated to phage proteins

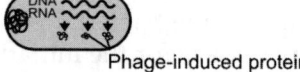

Phage-induced proteins

Step 4: Biosynthesis
Phage coat proteins, other protein components, and DNA are produced separately. Host DNA degraded

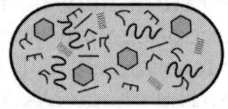

Fig. 2.54: Biosynthesis

4. **Maturation:** The phage DNA, head and tail protein are synthesized separately in the bacterial cell. The DNA is condensed into a compact polyhedron and 'packaged' into the head and finally, the tail structure is added. The process of assembly of the phage from its components is called 'maturation' (Fig. 2.55).

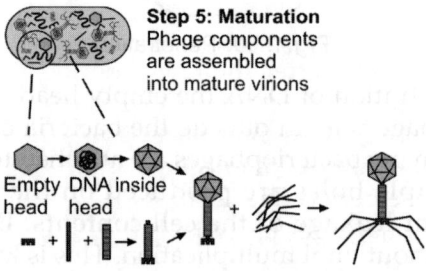

Step 5: Maturation
Phage components are assembled into mature virions

Empty DNA inside
head   head

Fig. 2.55: Maturation

5. **Release of progeny phage particles:** The release of progeny phage particles takes place by sudden explosion or bursting

(lysis) of the bacterial cell wall. Lysozymes synthesized within the cell causes the bacterial cell wall to break down and the newly produced Bacteriophages are released from the host cell. The released *bacteriophage* infects other susceptible bacterial cells. Each cycles of phage reproduction may require 20 to 60 minutes and a single phage infection may produce 200 of more progeny.

The sequence of events by the injection of the phage nucleic acid and release of newly synthesized virion is called 'replication cycle or viral multiplication'. The interval between the entry of the phage DNA into the bacterial cell and the appearance of the first infectious intracellular phage particle is known as the 'eclipse phase'. It represents the time required for the synthesis of the phage components and their assembly into mature phage particles (Fig. 2.56).

Step 6: Release
The bacterial cell lyses and releases many infective phage

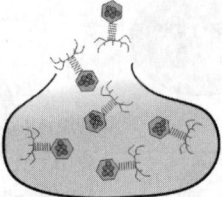

Fig. 2.56: Release

The interval between the infection of a bacterial cell and the first release of infectious phage particles is known as the 'latent period'. Immediately after the latent period, the number of phage particles released increases for a few minutes till the maximum number of daughter phage is reached. This period, during which the number of infectious phages released rises is known as the rise period (Fig. 2.56).

The yield of phage per bacterial cell is known as the 'burst size'.

ii. Lysogenic of Avirulent or Temperate Cycle

In contrast to virulent bacteriophages, temperate bacteriophages do not cause lysis of the host cell.

Following the entry into the host cell, the temperate phage nucleic acid becomes integrated with the bacterial chromosome. The integrated phage nucleic acid is known as the 'prophage'. The prophage behaves like a segment of the host chromosome and replicates synchronously in the bacterial cell. This is called 'lysogeny and bacterium that carries a prophage within its genome is called 'Lysogenic bacterium' (Fig. 2.57).

The prophage confers certain new properties on the lysogenic bacterium. This is known as 'lysogenic conversion' or phage conversion'. A Lysogenic bacterium is resistant to reinfection by

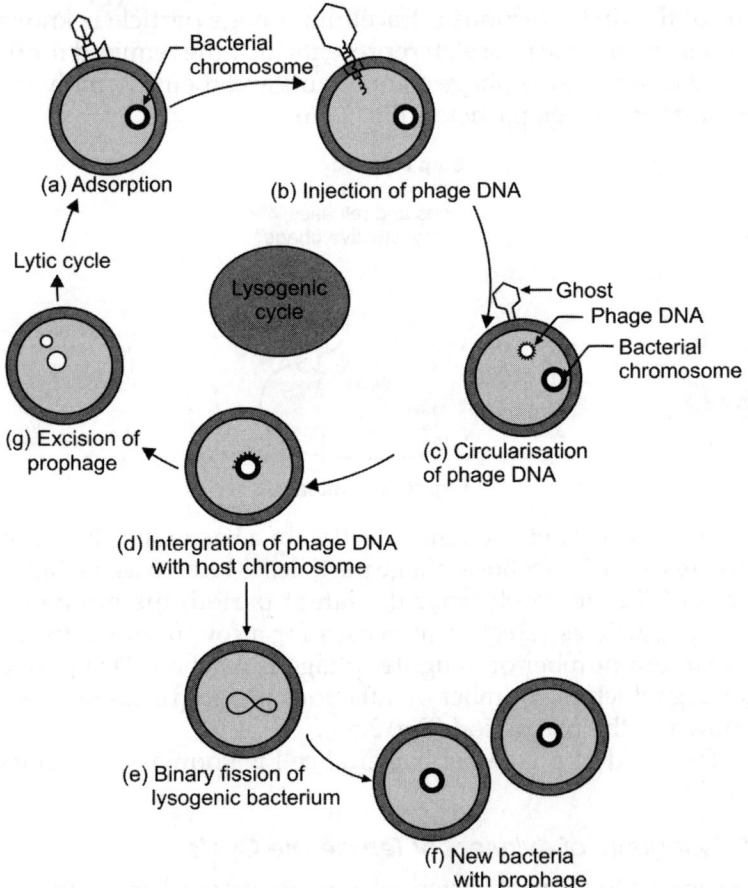

Fig. 2.57: Lysogenic life cycle of a bacteriophage

the same or related phages. This is known as 'super infection immunity. Every time the host cells machinery replicates the bacterial chromosome, it also replicates the prophage DNA. The prophage remains latent within the progeny cells. But due to spontaneous action of UV light or chemicals, the phage DNA separates from the bacterial cells. And lead to the excision of the phage DNA and to initiation of the lytic cycle. This is known as 'spontaneous induction of prophage'.

XXIII. ISOLATION AND IDENTIFICATION OF VIRUSES

Isolation and identification of virus can be accomplished by number of different methods but no single technique is satisfactory for all viruses or every kind of specimens.

The 1st step in laboratory identification of virus is the proper collection and care of specimens until susceptible animals, tissue cultures embryonated eggs or other appropriate media are inoculated. This includes making of specimen bacteria-free by filtration, differential centrifugation, or treatment with bactericidal agents. If a virus is present, characteristic antibodies, i.e. haemagglutination inhibiting, complement-fixing or neutralizing viral antibodies may be produced.

IMPORTANT STUDY QUESTIONS

1. Enlist the components of bacterial cell. Describe the flagella. (June 2011)

2. Write note on bacterial flagella. (Dec 2010)

3. Explain: Motility, Pathogenicity, and Virulence. (Dec 2010)

4. Describe type of bacteria on the basis of: (i) Nutritional requirement (ii) Temperature requirement. (Dec 2010)

5. Write note on Scanning Electron Microscopy. (Dec 2010)

6. Classify staining techniques. Discuss gram staining. (Dec 2010)

7. Enlist methods for isolation of bacteria. Discuss streak plate method. (Dec 2010, June 2011)

8. Classify the microorganisms. Differentiate the bacteria and viruses. (June 2011)

9. Enlist the various microscopic techniques. Give the three limitations of electron microscopy. (June 2011)

10. Differentiate gram-positive and gram-negative microorganisms. (June 2011, Dec 2011)

11. Enumerate the conditions requires for the growth of micro-organism. Draw a typical bacterial growth curve. (June 2011)

12. Classify the various media for bacterial growth. Discuss selective media. (June 2011)

13. Write a note on nutritional requirements of bacteria. (June 2011)

14. Classify organisms according to oxygen requirement. (Dec 2011)

15. Differentiate between light and electron microscopy. (Dec 2011)

16. How is specimen prepared, stained and viewed with electron microscopy? (Dec 2011)

17. Draw a neat labeled sketch of bacterial cell. (Dec 2011)

18. Differentiate between: (i) capsule and spore, (ii) selective and differential media. (Dec 2011)

19. Classify media. Write in detail about any one media used for cultivation of anaerobic organisms. (Dec 2011)

20. Enumerate and discuss various methods used for isolation of aerobes. (Dec 2011)

21. Write a note on spirochetes. (Dec 2011)

22. Discuss reproduction in fungi. (Dec 2011)

23. Define staining of microbes. Classify the types of staining.

24. Give detailed classification of bacteria.

25. Describe the structure of bacteria with functions of all structures.

26. Write a note on bacterial cell wall.

27. Write a note on bacterial structure internal to cell wall.

28. Write a note on bacterial structure external to cell wall.

29. Write a note on rickettsia and actinomycetes.

30. Discuss nutritional requirements of bacteria/virus.

31. Discuss in brief about growth cycle of bacteria.

32. Write in brief about reproduction of bacteria.

33. Write a note on cultivation of virus/bacteria.

3

Control of Microbes

I. Different Terms Employed to Control the Microorganisms

II. Ideal Properties of Growth Controlling Substances

III. Thermal Resistance of Microorganisms

IV. Factors Affecting the Thermal Destruction of the Microorganisms

V. Dynamics of Disinfection

VI. Factors Affecting the Disinfectant Action

VII. Major Group of Chemical Disinfectants

VIII. Methods of Sterilization

    A. Physical Methods

        1. Dry Heat Sterilization

        2. Moist Heat Sterilization

        3. Desiccation

        4. Osmotic Pressure

        5. Radiation Sterilization

    B. Chemical Methods

        1. Gaseous Sterilization

        2. Sterilization by Disinfectants

    C. Mechanical Methods

        1. Filtration

        2. Mechanism Involved in Filtration Sterilization

        3. Standardization and Testing of Filters

IX. Difference between Disinfection and Sterilization

X. Aseptic Techniques

XI. Precautions for Handling of Sterilization Equipment

XII. Evaluation of Disinfectants

    A. Test for Liquid Disinfectant

    B. Test for Semi-solid Disinfectant

C. Test for Solid Disinfectants
D. Tests on Aerial Disinfectants
XIII. Validation of Sterilization Method and Equipments
1. Physical Indicator
2. Chemical Indicator
3. Biological Indicator

I. DIFFERENT TERMS EMPLOYED TO CONTROL THE MICRO-ORGANISMS

The following terms are used to describe the process and substance which are employed to control the microorganisms.

Germicide (Microbicidal)

It is an agent that kills the growing forms of pathogenic bacteria (bacteria producing diseases) but not necessarily the resistant spore forms of germs.

Bactericide

It is an agent that kills bacteria.

Similarly, fungicide—kills fungi.

Virucide—kills viruses.

Sporicide—kills spores.

Bacteriostasis

It is the substance that prevents or retards the growth of bacteria.

Similarly, fungistatic—stops growth of fungi.

Microbiostatic—stops growth of microbes.

Antimicrobial Agent

It is the agent which interferes with growth and metabolism of microbes.

Sterilization

It is the process of destroying all forms of microbial life. Sterile means free of living microorganisms, or complete absence or destruction of all microorganisms.

Disinfectant

They are the substance that removes the infection potential of microorganism by destroying them but not necessarily the resistant spore forms. The term is commonly applied to substances used on inanimate objects.

Antiseptic

They are the substances that prevents sepsis, i.e. prevents the growth or action of microorganism either by destroying them or by inhibiting their growth and metabolism. It is usually associated with animate object, i.e. applied to the body.

Sanitizer

This is the agent that reduces the microbial population to safe levels as judged by public health requirements. Usually it is chemical agent that kills 99.9% of growing bacteria. It is commonly applied to inanimate objects and generally employed in daily care of equipment and utensils in dairies and food plants

II. IDEAL PROPERTIES OF GROWTH CONTROLLING SUBSTANCES

It is obvious that there is not a single chemical agent which is best for the control of microorganisms for any and all purposes. The specifications given below for such an ideal compound can be taken into consideration for the preparation of such new compounds.

Stability

There should not be any changes in the substance upon standing or if it is so, it should be minimal. It should not result in significant loss of germicidal action.

Antimicrobial activity

The capacity of the substance to kill or inhibit microorganism is the first requirement. The chemical at its lower concentration should exhibit its broad spectrum of antimicrobial activity.

Solubility

The agent must be soluble in water or other solvents to give its action for effective use.

Capacity to penetrate

The compound should have capacity to penetrate through surfaces; if it is not so then the germicidal action will be limited to the site of application. Sometimes, of course, only surface action is also the prime requirement.

Homogeneity

The preparation must be uniform in composition so that each active ingredient remains present in each application.

However, pure chemicals are uniform, but mixtures of materials may lack homogeneity.

Availability

The compound must be available in large quantities at the reasonable price.

Toxicity to microorganisms at room or body temperatures

The temperature of the compound used, should not be necessary to rise beyond the temperature of normal environment.

Nontoxicity to humans and other animals

Ideally, the agent should be lethal to the microorganisms but no injurious to humans and other animals.

Deodorizing ability

Deodorizing is the desirable attribute for the disinfectants. Ideally the disinfectant itself should either be odorless or should have a pleasant smell.

Detergent capacities

A disinfectant which is also a detergent (cleansing agent) will provide the two objectives. The cleansing action improves the effectiveness of the disinfectants.

Non-combination with extraneous organic materials

Most disinfectants have affinity for proteins or other organic material. So, when this organic material is present besides that of the microbial cells, only a little disinfectant also, if available, will give its action against the microorganisms.

Noncorroding and bonstaining

It should not rust or disfigure the metals and also it should not stain or damage the fabrics.

III. THERMAL RESISTANCE OF MICROORGANISMS

The microorganisms show different resistance to different methods of sterilization. The degree of resistance differs with the specific microorganism, particularly with the spores of microorganisms which are more resistant than the vegetative forms of the organism. Therefore, before selecting any method of sterilization, it must be kept in mind that the method and its conditions must be lethal to the resistant spores. For that the following points should be taken into consideration:

1. **Thermal death time:** It may be defined as the time required to kill a specific type of microorganisms at a given temperature under specific conditions. It depends on many factors like temperature, pH, presence of bactericide, number of contaminating microorganisms, their resistance to heat, etc. Table 3.1 shows approximate values of thermal death times of different spores to moist heat and dry heat.

Table 3.1: Approximate thermal death times of different spores

Organisms	Time in minutes					
	Moist heat			Dry heat		
Bacillus anthracis	5–15	–	–	–	180	–
Clostridium welchii	5–15	–	–	50	5	–
Clostridium tetani	5–15	–	–	–	15	–
Clostridium botulinum	330	90	10	120	60	15
Soil bacillus	>1020	120	6	–	–	15

From the above table it is seen that there is a considerable variation in thermal death time between different types of bacterial spores. Therefore, an adequate safety margin should be kept to kill the most resistant species of microorganisms and spores expected to be present by exceeding temperature and time of most of the spores.

2. **Death rate of microorganisms:** There is no direct method to determine when the sterility will be achieved. It is because the reason that shortly before the sterility is reached, the number of living microorganisms is too small. Thus the accurate determination of it becomes impossible due to very high errors in taking the samples. The reliable approach is to plot a graph between the Log survivals of microorganisms against time of exposure.

3. **Decimal reduction time (D value):** It is defined as the time in minutes required reducing the number of viable

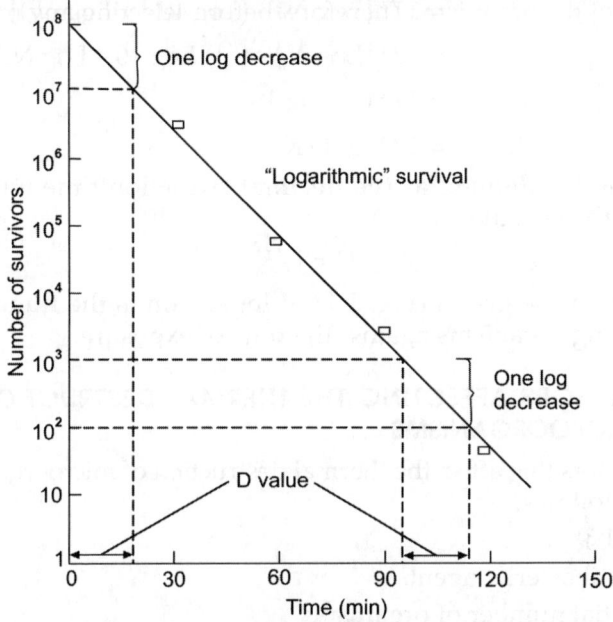

Fig. 3.1: Graph illustrating the concept of decimal reduction time (*D* value)

organisms by 90%. It is one of the functions to indicate the efficiency of sterilization process.

The order of death of microorganisms can be calculated from the equation:

$$K = 1/t \, (\text{Log } N_0 - \text{Log } N) \qquad \qquad ... (3.1)$$

Where,

K = constant which depends on organism, temperature and medium

t = time of exposure in minutes

N_0 = Number of organisms viable at the beginning of time interval

N = Number of organisms viable at the end of the time interval

It was noted that after 90% reduction in microorganisms the following equation was obtained:

$$K = 1/t \, (\text{Log } N_0 - \text{Log } 0.1 \, N_0)$$
$$= 1/t \, (\text{Log } N_0 - \text{Log } 10^{-1} \, N_0)$$

$$= 1/t \ [\text{Log } N_0 - (\text{Log } 10^{-1} + \text{Log } N_0)]$$
$$= 1/t \ [\text{Log } N_0 - (-1) \ \text{Log } 10 - \text{Log } N_0]$$
$$= 1/t \ (1) \ \text{Log } 10$$
$$= 1/t \ t = 1/K$$

Time t is defined as the decimal reduction time which is called the D value.

$$D = 1/K$$

K from the graph (Fig. 3.1) of logarithm is the number of surviving organisms against the time of exposure.

IV. FACTORS AFFECTING THE THERMAL DESTRUCTION OF MICROORGANISMS

The factors that affect the thermal destruction of microorganisms are as follows:

1. pH
2. Antibacterial agents
3. Initial number of organisms
4. Inhibitory medicaments
5. Protective substances
6. The inactivation factor of the process

1. **pH:** The most of all microorganisms are resistant to heat at the pH of 6–8. So, acidic or alkaline solutions are easier to sterilize. There are some substances such as alkaloidal salts which act as buffers for acidic or alkaline pH may be used for maintaining the stability. Such condition helps in the sterilization of an injection.

2. **Antibacterial agents:** The addition of antibacterial agent in injections like form can decrease the sterilization temperature from 115° to 100°C. This is very useful for the sterilization of thermolabile substances. This method of sterilization is commonly called as *Sterilization by heating with bactericide.*

3. **Initial number of organisms:** When certain numbers of organisms are heated at a lethal temperature, the organisms are not killed all at once, but they are killed gradually as the exposure is prolonged. If certain fraction of initial number is destroyed in a particular time interval then the

same fraction will be destroyed in the next (succeeding) interval of time. This will continue till all the organisms are killed and the preparation is sterilized. If the initial numbers of organisms are less, then the time required for sterilization will also be less.

Therefore, while preparing the solutions, every precaution should be taken to eliminate the entry of microorganisms. Also as far as possible, thoroughly cleaned containers and equipment's should be used.

4. **Inhibitory medicaments:** There are certain medicaments which when prepared into solution form, are harmful to microorganisms. This is because of pH in certain cases or it may be due to the toxic effect of the medicaments itself. Although, some of the non-sporing microorganisms, for, e.g. *Staphylococcus aureus* are killed within 24 hours at room temperature by a number of medicaments in their usual strength, but their spores are not killed unless they are heated to sterilizing conditions of time and temperature. So there are only very few injections, which can be safely regarded as self-sterilizing material.

5. **Protective substances:** The microorganisms are not killed easily in the media containing high concentrations of organic substances such as proteins and carbohydrates. The reason is not known clearly but it is believed that protein forms a protective coat on the cells. Most of the injections which contain the protein are thermolabile. So, they cannot be sterilized by the use of heat. Hence, they do not create much problem. But this effect is found in injections containing thermostable carbohydrates such as dextrose which is used in high concentration.

But it is observed that any increase in resistance of organisms is overcome by normal sterilizing conditions. These types of problems are more important in case of sterilization of glass wares and equipment such as tubes, syringes, containers, etc. because they are not thoroughly cleaned after use for proteins like blood or blood products and carbohydrates like dextrose. The reason is because some of the microorganisms may remain hidden inside the equipment and protected from steam. So, it is desirable that the glasswares and equipment's should be thoroughly cleaned before sterilization.

6. **The inactivation factor of the process:** The inactivation factor means the degree to which the viable population of organism is decreased. It is obtained by dividing the initial viable count by the final viable count

$$\text{Inactivation factor} = 10t/D$$

Where,

t = Exposure time in minutes

D = Decimal reduction time for the same temperature and condition

V. DYNAMICS OF DISINFECTION

Action rates of antimicrobial chemicals: *Watson* derived mathematical expressions from *Chick's* data and showed that the reaction rate could be expressed in the same form as a first order chemical reaction. The determinant will be the numbers of cells in the culture. Interpretation of these types of results is based on the theoretical mechanisms and they are called mechanistic theories.

The resulting expression is:

$$K = \text{Log } (a/a - x)t^{-1}$$

Where,

K is the rate constant; t is the time of contact before sample is removed; a is the initial number of bacteria in the culture $a - x$ is the number of organisms in the same volume after exposure for time t

When death occurs at the faster rate, the plot is a straight line; hence the term logarithmic order of death is often used to describe this type of death rate.

VI. FACTORS AFFECTING THE DISINFECTANT ACTION

Some of the main factors affecting disinfectant action are:

1. Time of contact
2. Concentration of disinfectant
3. Temperature
4. The type of organism present, its numbers and condition

5. The presence of organic matter and other inactivators
6. Hydrogen ion concentration
7. Surface tension
8. The formulation of the disinfectant
9. The chemical structure of the disinfectant
10. The nature of surface to be disinfect
11. Potentiation, synergism and antagonism of disinfectants

1. **Time of contact:** A plot of viable count of bacterial population against time when the population is subjected to lethal environment will give death/mortality curve. It follows unimolecular reaction. The principle of first order kinetics would be applied to disinfectant effect and the velocity constant/rate constant, 'k', is the measure of efficiency of disinfectant.

$$K = \frac{1}{t} \text{Log} \frac{B}{b}$$

Where,

t = Time for the viable count to fall from B to b

B = Initial number of organisms

b = Final number of organisms

The survivor v/s time curve is not constant, its shape being influenced by a number of factors, especially the concentration of disinfectant being used (Fig. 3.2).

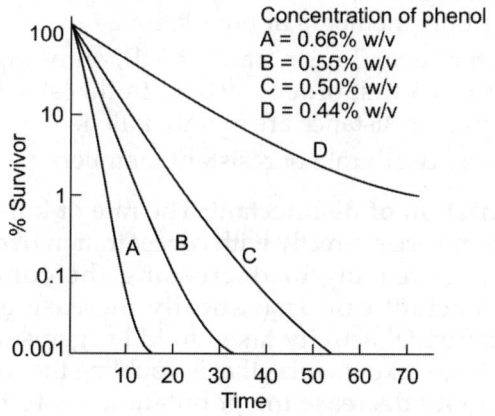

Fig. 3.2: Effect of concentration of phenol on survivor v/s time curves of *E.coli*

Main three types of death curve are shown in disinfection processes which are shown in Fig. 3.3.

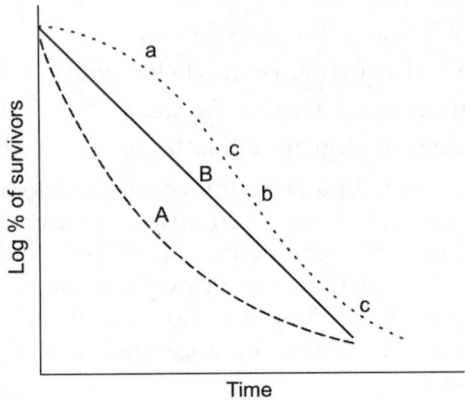

Fig. 3.3: Main types of death curves shown in disinfection processes

Where,

Curve A shows that disinfection process obeying first order kinetic low (only sometimes obtained)

Curve B, often obtained with high concentrations of disinfectant.

Curve C shows sigmoid curve which is usually obtained

The process is divided in three stages

a. Slow initial kill, which is mainly seen for sensitive or susceptible members of population.

b. A faster 'near-linear' rate of kill, showing a similar pattern to a first order reaction. In this stage, organism of average resistance are mainly killed.

c. A slower death rate of resistant members.

2. **Concentration of disinfectant:** The rate of kill of bacterial population varies directly with concentration of disinfectant. Slightly increasing or decreasing the concentration of disinfectant can dramatically increase or decrease the bactericidal activity taken to kill organism at a given temperature is exponential, that is doubling the concentration considerably decrease the population, more than halves the rate, if the concentration exponent is greater than 1.

It is expressed by the formula:

$$C^n t = a \text{ constant } (k)$$

Where,

C = concentration

n = concentration exponent or dilution co-efficient for the disinfectant

t = death time

The equation can also be written as:

$$n \text{ Log } C + \text{Log } t = a \text{ constant } (k)$$

Therefore, if the graph is plotted of Log t against Log C, a straight line is usually obtained and the slope of the line is the concentration exponent (Fig. 3.4).

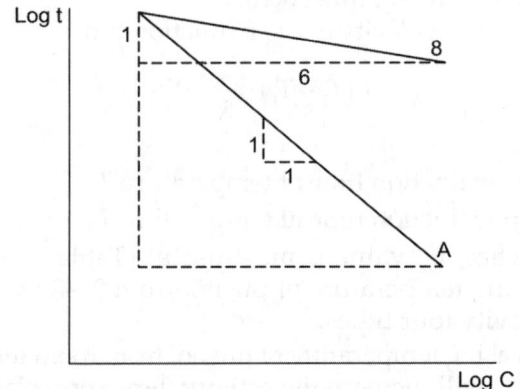

Fig. 3.4: Graphical determination of concentration exponent of disinfectant

The value of n may be obtained graphically of by substitution in the equation:

$$n = \frac{\text{Log } t_2 - \text{Log } t_1}{\text{Log } C_1 - \text{Log } C_2}$$

Where,

t_1 = death time with disinfectant concentration

$C_1 t_2$ = death time with disinfectant concentration C_2

The value of n is affected by the factors which influence disinfection, i.e. temperature, type of organism, environmental factors and the formulations.

3. **Temperature:** Temperature is directly proportional to bactericidal activity. As the temperature increases, bactericidal activity also increases. The relationship between the temperature and velocity of reaction is being shown in figure and may be expressed by equation:

$$\theta(T_2 - T_1) = \frac{k_2}{k_1}$$

Where,

k_1 = extinction time at temperature T_1

k_2 = extinction time at temperature T_2

θ = temperature coefficient

Extinction time is the time at which no living cells can be detected in the sample taken.

The reaction velocity $k \propto 1/$Extinction time

$$\theta(T_2 - T_1) = \frac{k_2}{k_1} = \frac{t_1}{t_2}$$

Where,

t_1 = extinction time at temperature T_1

t_2 = extinction time at temperature T_2

In practice, θ^{10} value is most useful (Table 3.2). Effect of increasing temperature of phenol from 20–30°C, increases the activity four times.

Increasing temperature of phenol from room temperature to 100°C will increase the activity very appreciably and in addition, higher temperatures have an adverse effect on growth of microorganism (Fig. 3.5).

Table 3.2: Values of θ for common bactericides

Disinfectant	θ (20°C)	θ^{10}
Phenol	1.15	4.0
o-cresol	1.18	5.1
p-cresol	1.19	5.8
Resorcinol	1.22	7.1
Ethylene glycol	1.34	18.0
n-butanol	1.41	31.0
Ethanol	1.46	43
Ethylene glycol monoethyl ether	1.76	291

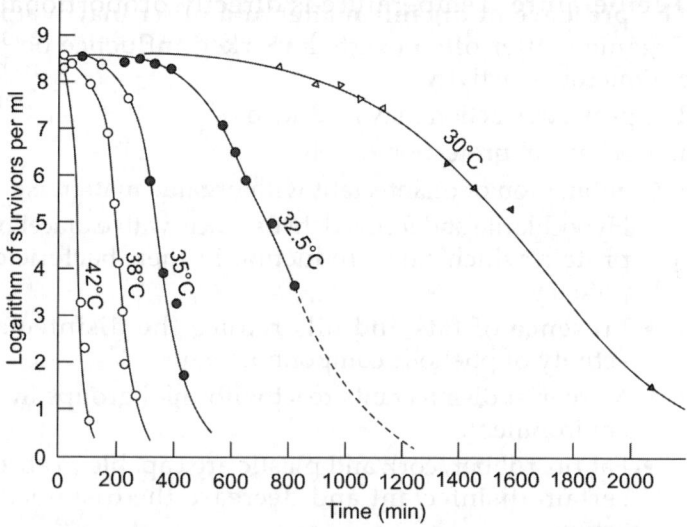

Fig. 3.5: Increase in temperature decreases bacterial survival when the concentration of disinfectant remains constant

4. **The type of organism present, its numbers and condition:**
   The type of organism, number and the condition of the organisms all affect the disinfection process. The most vegetative bacteria, with the exceptions of acid–fast bacilli, are rapidly killed by most chemical disinfectants. Apart from acid-fast bacilli many *Pseudomonas* species are highly resistant to antimicrobial substances. Bacterial spores are difficult to destroy but some aldehydes are sporicidal. Aldehydes and halogens together with β-propiolactone are most active virucides. Antifungal activity varies considerably and many disinfectants have a limited spectrum of activity.

   The success of disinfection is often dependent on the degree of initial concentration. A large number of microorganisms initially often lead to longer disinfection times or greater concentrations of disinfectant are required to achieve a satisfactory killing effect. Resistance of microorganisms varies with their age and conditions under which they are grown. In any description of disinfectant action the inoculums size, age, and past history should be stated.

5. The presence of organic matter and other inactivators: Organic matter often exerts a marked influence on the antimicrobial activity.

The protective action may be due to

a. Mechanical protection of cell

b. Combination of disinfectant with organic matter, e.g.

- Hypochlorite and formaldehyde reacts with extracellular protein which cause reduction in their bactericidal potency.
- Presence of fats and oils reduce the disinfectant activity of phenolic compound.
- Mercurial disinfectants react with thiol groups in the environment.
- Fabric, rubber, cork and plastic are capable to absorb certain disinfectant and decrease the disinfectant action.

6. Hydrogen ion concentration (pH): pH during the disinfectant process affects:

1. Rate of growth of microorganism.

2. Degree of ionization of antimicrobial substance and therefore its potency.

3. Absorption of antimicrobial substance at cell surface.

   The optimum pH for the bacterial growth is in the range of 6 to 7.

4. Outside this range, growth may be inhibited to some extent, e.g.

   - Phenol, benzoic acid, salicylic acid are most effective in acidic pH in its unionized form.
   - Most acridine compound in which cation is most active they are used for wounds and skin infection are well ionized at pH 7.
   - Basic dyes such as crystal violet, brilliant green and the cationic surfactant the activity is increased by increasing pH.

7. Surface tension: Many surface active compound and mainly cationic quaternary ammonium compounds are highly bactericidal. Small amount of anionic surfactant is added to phenol, it reduces the extinction time because of the reduction of surface tension and therefore faster penetration of bacteria by the phenolic solution. Soap can be used. More soap is added, the lower the surface tension and lower the extinction time until the soap concentration is equivalent to the critical concentration for micelle formation (CMC). In excess of this concentration the surface tension remains almost constant, but the extinction time increases due to phenol leaving the aqueous phase and entering the interior of micelles (Fig. 3.6).

8. **The formulation of the disinfectant:** Correct formulation is important for the effective use of disinfectant because it affects the penetration power and therefore its effectiveness. Often disinfectant may be formulated in either aqueous solution or in 70% alcohol, e.g.

   • Chlorhexidine and some quaternary ammonium compound are formulated as alcoholic formulation. Therefore penetration power in increased and antimicrobial activity is increased

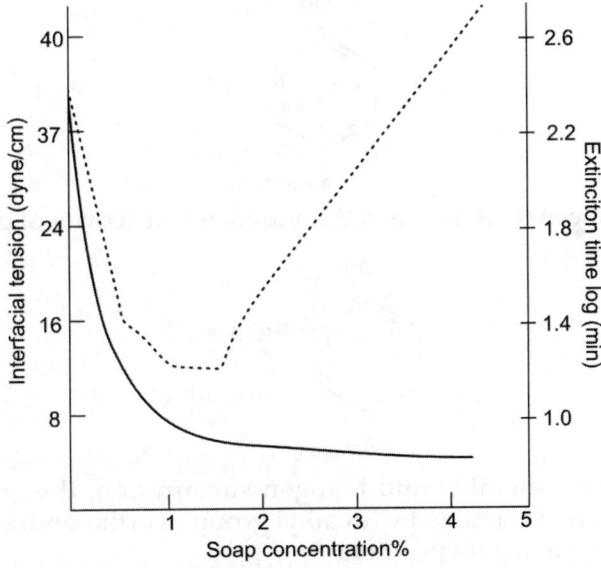

Fig. 3.6: Relation between extinction time of *E. coli* and the interfacial tension of phenol/soap mixtures

- Phenols have low solubility in water therefore concentrated solution in water or emulsion are prepared using soaps and colloids
- Iodine is insoluble in water and it is dissolved in alcohol, potassium iodide solution or solution of surface active agent. The presence of suitable surfactant can moderate the staining and corrosive property of the iodine and therefore increases the stability of preparation.
- Non-ionic surfactants of the tween series have been shown to reduce the activity of preservatives especially methyl and propyl p-hydroxybenzoate, a factor must be taken in mind during the formulation of pharmaceutical product.

9. **The chemical structure of the disinfectant:** Substitution of an alkyl chain up to six carbon length in para-position to the phenolic –OH group increases the activity. Substitution of alkyl chain more than six carbons decreases water solubility and therefore decreases activity. Straight alkyl chain gives greater activity than branched alkyl chain.

Halogenation increases the antimicrobial activity of phenol.

With both alkyl and halogen substitution, the greatest activity is obtained with alkyl group in ortho position and halogen in para position.

Nitration increases antimicrobial activity and systematic toxicity.

OH

Nitro group

10. **The nature of the surface to be disinfected:** Bactericides work effectively on hard, clean, impenetrable surfaces. Microorganisms are inaccessible to disinfectant when they are present in uneven, porous or cracked surfaces. Aqueous environment is required for disinfection organic and oily liquids. Dried films of blood, pus, sputum impact the penetration of disinfectant. Disinfectant should not react adversely with the surface; it should not leave the detrimental residual effect which cannot be easily eliminated. Disinfectant if used for living tissues, it should not be toxic to underlying cells.

11. **Potentiating, synergism and antagonism of disinfectants:** Potentiating of disinfectant (mainly by inactive substances) leads to enhanced antimicrobial activity. Synergistic effects are often shown by two antimicrobial agents working together and either giving an increased activity (more than their additive effect) or an increased spectrum of activity (i.e. lethal to a greater range of organisms). Antagonism leads to decreased antimicrobial activity and use of antagonists is made of antagonists in the elimination of antimicrobial properties of materials which are being tested by sterility (Table 3.3).

VII. MAJOR GROUP OF CHEMICAL DISINFECTANTS

Phenol and Phenolic Compound

Phenol had been used successfully in the 1880s by *Joseph Lister*, a surgeon, to reduce infection of surgical incisions and surgical wounds. He also developed the practice of spraying phenol into the operating room area to control infection. Phenol is the standard against which other disinfectants of a similar chemical structure are compared to determine their antimicrobial activity. The procedure used is called the phenol-coefficient technique. This technique is described later in this chapter.

Table 3.3: Potentiating and antagonism of disinfectants

Disinfectant	Potentiating agent	Antagonist
Benzalkonium chloride	Low concentrations of non-ionic surfactants	
Chlorhexidine diacetate		
p-Hydroxybenzoates	Polysorbate 80	
Chlorine compounds	Bromine or iodine compounds	
Halogens		Sodium thiosulphate
Quaternary ammonium compounds		Anionic agents, e.g. lubrol W+, lecithin, soaps, milk
Mercurials and arsenicals		Thioglycolic acid, sulphhydryl compounds

Phenol and phenolic compounds are very effective disinfectants. A 5 % aqueous solution of phenol rapidly kills the vegetative cells of microorganisms, but spores are much more resistant. Many derivatives of phenol were found to have antimicrobial activity. The chemical structures of phenol and few phenol derivatives are shown below:

Phenol   o-cresol   m-cresol

Hexylresorcinol   Hexachlorophene

p-cresol   p-phenylphenol

Antimicrobial activity is enhanced by the addition of chemical substitutions in the phenol ring structure as shown in Table 3.4.

Table 3.4: Microbial action of phenol derivatives (numerical in table shows phenol coefficients at 37°C)

Name of phenol derivative	Salmonella typhi	Staphylococcus aureus	Mycobacterium tuberculosis	Candida albicans
Phenol	1.0	1.0	1.0	1.0
o-cresol	2.3	2.3	2.0	2.0
m-cresol	2.3	2.3	2.0	2.0
p-cresol	2.3	2.3	2.0	2.0
4-Ethylphenol	6.3	6.3	6.7	7.8

The higher the value, the greater the antimicrobial activity. The antimicrobial activity of phenolic is reduced at an alkaline pH and by organic material. Low temperatures and the presence of soap also reduce antimicrobial activity.

Mode of action

Exposure of microbial cells to phenolic compounds produces a variety of effects. Depending upon the concentration of the phenolic compound to which microbial cells were exposed, the results like, disruption of cells, precipitation of cell protein, inactivation of enzymes and leakage of amino acids from cells have been obtained. Although the specific mode of action is not clear, the lethal effect is associated with physical damage to the membrane structure in the cell surface, which initiates further deterioration.

Practical application

1. Hexylresorcinol, a derivative of phenol, is marketed in the solution of glycerin in water. It is strong surface tension reluctant, which may account in part for its high bactericidal activity. Its preparations are also employed as general antiseptics.

2. Phenolic substances may be either bactericidal or bacteriostatic, depending upon the concentration used.

3. Bacterial spores and viruses are more resistant than the vegetative cells.

4. Some phenolics are highly fungicidal.

5. The antimicrobial activity of aqueous solutions of pure crystalline phenol from 2 to 5% can be employed to disinfect materials such as sputum, urine, feces and contaminated instruments or utensils. Solutions of pure phenol have limited application.

6. The derivatives of phenol diluted in detergents or some other carrier are used in many commercial antiseptic and disinfectant preparations.

Alcohols

Ethyl alcohol, in concentrations between 50 and 90%, is effective against vegetative or non-spore forming cells. For practical application a 70% concentration of alcohol is generally used. Ethyl alcohol cannot produce a sterile condition. Concentrations which are effective against vegetative cells are practically inert against bacterial spores.

Sykes notes that there is one record of survival of anthrax spores in alcohol for 20 years and another one of the *Bacillus subtilis* for 9 years.

Methyl alcohol is less bactericidal than ethyl alcohol; but it is highly poisonous. Even the fumes of this compound may produce permanent injury to the eyes, and it is generally employed for destruction of microorganisms. The higher alcohols—propyl, butyl, amyl and others are more germicidal than ethyl alcohol. In fact, there is a progressive increase in germicidal power as the molecular weight of alcohols increases (Table 3.5).

Table 3.5: Result analysis of germicidal power of microorganism as per molecular weight of alcohol

Alcohol	Phenol-coefficient	
	Against Salmonella typhi	Against Staphylococcus aureus
Methyl	0.026	0.03
Ethyl	0.04	0.039
n-Propyl	0.102	0.082
Isopropyl	0.064	0.054
n-Butyl	0.273	0.22
n-Amyl	0.78	0.63

Mode of action

Alcohols are protein denaturants, and this property accounts for their antimicrobial activity. Alcohols are also solvents for lipids, and hence, they may damage lipid complexes in the cell membrane. They are also dehydrating agents. This may ineffective for absolute alcohols on dry cells. They serves dehydration occurring under these conditions would result in a bacteriostatic condition. Some of the effectiveness of alcohol can also cause cleansing or detergent action which results in mechanical removal of microorganisms.

Practical applications

1. Alcohol is effective in reducing the microbial flora of skin and for the disinfection of clinical and oral thermometers.
2. Alcohol concentrations above 60% are effective against viruses; however, the effectiveness is influenced considerable by the amount of extraneous protein material in the mixture. The extraneous protein reacts with the alcohol and thus protects the virus.

Halogens

Iodine

Iodine is one of the oldest and most effective germicidal agents. It has been in the use for more than a century. It has been recognized by the U.S. Pharmacopoeia in 1830. Pure iodine is bluish-black crystalline element having a metallic luster.

It is only slightly soluble in water but readily soluble in alcohol and aqueous solutions of potassium or sodium iodide. It is traditionally used as a germicidal agent as 'tincture of iodine'. Iodine is also used in the form of substances known as 'iodophors'. They are mixtures of iodine with surface active agents which act as carriers and solubilizers for the iodine. They possess the germicidal characteristics of iodine and have the additional advantages of non-staining and low irritant properties.

Mode of action

The mechanisms by which iodine exert their antimicrobial activity is not properly understood. Iodine is an oxidizing agent and by that shows its antimicrobial action. Oxidizing agents can irreversibly oxidize and thus inactivate essential metabolic compounds such as proteins with sulfhydryl groups. It has been also observed that the action may involve the halogen action of tyrosine units of enzymes and other cellular proteins requiring tyrosine for activity.

Practical application

1. Iodine is highly effective bactericidal agent and it is a unique, i.e. it is effective against all kinds of bacteria
2. Iodine also possesses sporicidal activity but the rate at which the spores are killed is markedly influenced by the conditions upon which they are exposed.
3. It is highly fungicidal and is to some extent virucidal.
4. Iodine solutions are chiefly used for the disinfection of skin. Iodine preparation is also effective for reduction of the microbial flora of the skin.
5. Iodine preparations are effective for other purposes such as disinfection of water, disinfection of air, and sanitization of food utensils.

Chlorine and chlorine compounds

Chlorine, either in the form of gas or in the combination with certain chemicals, is one of the best widely used disinfectants. The compressed gas in liquid form is almost universally employed for the purification of municipal water supplies. Chlorine gas is difficult to handle unless special equipment is available to dispense it. So, its usefulness in the gaseous form is limited to large-scale operations, e.g. in water purification plants.

There are many chlorine compounds available which can be handled more conveniently than free chlorine and it is equally effective as disinfectants. One of the compounds in this category is the 'hypochlorites', e.g. calcium hypochlorite $Ca(OCl)_2$ also known as chlorinated lime, sodium hypochlorite $NaOCl$, etc. Another category of chlorine compounds used as disinfectants is 'chloramines' which are also used as sanitizing agents and antiseptics. Chemically they are characterized that one or more of the hydrogen atoms in an amino group of a compound are replaced by chlorine. Chloramines are more stable than that of hypochlorites in terms of prolonged release of chlorine.

Mode of action

The antimicrobial action of chlorine and its compounds comes through the hypochlorous acid which is formed when free chlorine is added to water:

$$Cl_2 + H_2O \rightarrow HCl + HClO \text{ (hypochlorous acid)}$$

Similarly, hypochlorites and chloramines undergo hydrolysis, with the formation of hypochlorous acid. The formed hypochlorous acid is further decomposed.

$$HClO \rightarrow O + HCl \text{ (formed from chlorine, hypochlorites and chloramines)}$$

The oxygen released in this reaction (nascent oxygen) is a strong oxidizing agent, and through its action on microorganism's cellular constituents they are destroyed. The killing of microorganisms by chlorine and its compounds is also because of direct combination of chlorine with proteins of the cell membranes and enzymes.

Practical application

1. Hypochlorite is used to reduce the incidence of childbed fever.
2. Medical students can use this hypochlorite solution for washing their hands and soak them before examining patients.
3. Chlorine compounds are very widely used to control the microorganisms mainly, for water treatment, in the food industry, for domestic uses and in medicine.

4. Products containing calcium hypochlorite are used for sanitizing dairy equipment and eating utensils in restaurants.

5. Solution of sodium hypochlorite of 1% concentration is used for personal hygiene and as a household disinfectant; higher concentrations of 5 to 12% are also employed as household bleaches, disinfectants, for sanitizing agents in dairy and food processing establishments.

6. Chlorine compounds have been used to disinfect open wounds, to treat athlete's foot, to treat other infections and as general disinfectant.

Heavy Metals and their Compounds

Most of the heavy metals either alone or in combination with certain compounds, exert a detrimental effect upon micro-organisms. The most effective are mercury, silver and copper. Examples of these compounds are summarized as below:

Mode of action

Heavy metals and their compounds act antimicrobially by combining with cellular proteins and make them inactivated.

$$\text{Enzyme} \begin{matrix} SH \\ \\ SH \end{matrix} + HgCl_2 \longrightarrow \text{Enzyme} \begin{matrix} S \\ Hg + 2HCl \\ S \end{matrix}$$

Active enzyme Mercuric chloride   Inactive enzyme

High concentrations of salts of heavy metals like mercury, copper and silver coagulate cytoplasmic proteins, resulting in damage or death of the cell.

Mercury (Inorganic compound)

Examples of these compounds include Mercuric chloride, Mercurous chloride, Mercuric oxide, Ammoniated mercury.

Application

1. They are bactericidal in dilutions of 1:1000.

2. It is limited in use because of its corrosive action, high toxicity to animals, and reduction of effectiveness in presence of organic material.

3. They are insoluble and used in ointments as antiseptics

Organic compound

Example includes Mercurochrome, Metaphen, Merthiolate, Mercresin.

Application

1. They are less irritating and less toxic than the inorganic mercury compound.
2. They are employed as antiseptics on cutaneous and mucosal surfaces.
3. They may be bactericidal or bacteriostatic.

Silver (colloidal silver compounds)

Example includes Silver nitrate, Silver lactate, Silver picrate.

Application

1. It consist of protein in combination with metallic silver or silver oxide and used as an antiseptics.
2. They possess bacteriostatic or bactericidal effect.
3. The eyes of newborns are treated with a few drops of 1% silver nitrate solution to prevent ophthalmia neonatorum, a gonococcal infection of eyes.

Copper

Example includes Copper sulfate.

Application

1. They are much more effective against algae and molds than bacteria.
2. They are used in swimming pools and open water reservoirs.
3. They are used in the form of Bordeaux mixture as a fungicide for prevention of certain plant diseases.

Dyes

Two classes of dye compounds are known for their antimicrobial properties

1. Triphenylmethane
2. Acridine dyes

Triphenylmethane

Examples of these dyes are malachite green, brilliant green and crystal violet. The gram-positive organisms are more susceptible to lower concentrations of these compounds than the gram-negative ones.

Example

1. Crystal violet will inhibit *gram-positive cocci* at a dilution of 1:2,000,000 to 1:3,000,000. And 10 times of this concentration is required to inhibit *E. coli.*
2. *Staphylococcus aureus* is inhibited by malachite green at a concentration of 1:1,000,000, whereas the concentration of about 1:30,000 is required to inhibit *E. coli.*

Mode of action

The mode of action of triphenylmethane dyes is uncertain, but there is speculation that they exert their inhibitory effect by interfering with cellular oxidation process.

Practical application

1. Certain media can be added with dyes such as crystal violet, brilliant green, or malachite green to inhibit *gram-positive bacteria*.
2. Media of this kind is used extensively in public health microbiology
3. Susceptibility to various dyes can also be used for identification of bacteria
4. Crystal violet has also been used as a fungicide. A concentration of 1:10,000 is lethal for Monilia and Torula and a concentration of 1:1,000,000 is inhibitory.

Acridine dyes

Two examples of acridine derived dyes are:

1. Acriflavine
2. Tryptoflavine

These compounds exhibit selective inhibition against bacteria, particularly *Staphylococci* and *Gonococci*. *Gonococci* are inhibited by tryptoflavine in dilutions of 1:1,00,00,000. They possess antifungal activity. In some extent they are used for the treatment of burns, wounds and also for ophthalmic application and bladder irrigation.

Synthetic Detergents

Surface tension depressant or wetting agents can be employed primarily for cleansing surfaces are called as 'detergents'. Soap is an example. However, soap is a poor detergent in hard water. For this reason many new more efficient cleansing agents have been developed, called 'surfactants' or 'synthetic detergents', which are superior to soap.

Chemically detergents are classified as below:

1. Those which ionize with the detergent property and remains in the anion are referred to as anionic detergents, e.g. soap, sodium lauryl sulphate
2. Those which ionize with detergent property and remains in the cation are referred to as cationic detergents, e.g. cetylpyridinium chloride.
3. The third category of detergent is 'nonionic', i.e. they do not ionize. However, these substances do not possess significant antimicrobial activity.

Practical application

They are extensively used in laundries and dish washing powders, shampoos and other washing preparations. Some are also highly bactericidal.

Mode of action

They reduce surface tension and thereby increase wetting power of the water in which they are dissolved. Soapy water has ability to emulsify and disperse the oil and the dirt. The microorganism may become enmeshed in the soap lather and are removed by the rinse water.

Quarternary Ammonium Compounds

Most compounds of the germicidal cationic detergent class are 'quarternary ammonium salts'. The bactericidal power of the quarternaries is exceptionally high against *gram-positive bacteria*, and they are also quite active against *gram-negative organisms*. Bactericidal concentrations range from dilutions of one part in little thousand to one part in several hundred thousand. It possesses the bacteriostatic action far beyond their bactericidal concentration. For example, the limit of bactericidal action for a given compound may be at a dilution of 1:30,000 yet it may be bacteriostatic in dilutions as high as 1:200,000. Quaternaries have been shown to be fungicidal as well as destructive to certain of the pathogenic protozoa. Viruses appear to be more resistant than bacteria and fungi.

Mode of action

A variety of damaging effects have been observed by the use of quaternaries. This includes denaturation of proteins, interference with glycolysis and membrane damage. The most likely site of the damage to the cell is the cytoplasmic membrane; the quaternaries alter the vital permeability features of this cell structure.

Practical application

The combined properties of germicidal activity and detergent action, plus such other features like low toxicity, high solubility in water, stability in solution and non-corrosiveness, makes the quaternary compounds for the use as a disinfectants and sanitizing agents. They are used as skin disinfectants, as a preservative in ophthalmic solutions and in cosmetic preparations. They are widely used for control of micro-organisms on floors, walls, and other surfaces in hospitals, nursing homes and other public places.

They are used to sanitize the food and beverage utensils in restaurants as well as surfaces and certain equipment in food processing plants. Other applications are to be found in the dairy, egg, and fishing industries to control the microbial growth on the surfaces of equipment and the environment in general.

Aldehydes

Among the various aldehydes among the class of chemicals, several of the low-molecular-weight compounds are anti-microbial. Two of the most effective are formaldehyde and glutaraldehyde, both are highly microbicidal and both possess the ability to kill spores.

Formaldehyde

It is the simplest compound in the aldehydes series. It is a gas that is stable only in high concentrations and at elevated temperatures. At room temperature it polymerizes, forming a solid substance. Formaldehyde is also marketed in aqueous solution as formalin, which contains 37 to 40% formaldehyde. The fumes of formaldehyde are noxious. They are irritating to tissues and eyes.

Mode of action

It is an extremely reactive chemical. It combines readily with vital organic nitrogen compounds such as proteins and nucleic acids. It is likely that interaction of formaldehyde with these cellular substances accounts for its antimicrobial action.

Practical application

1. Formaldehyde in the solution form is useful for sterilization of certain instruments.
2. In the gaseous form it can be used for disinfection and sterilization of enclosed areas.
3. Vaporization of formaldehyde from either of these sources into an enclosed area for an adequate time will cause sterilization, vegetative cells being killed more quickly than spores.

Glutaraldehyde

It is a saturated dialdehyde. A 2% solution of this chemical agent exhibits a wide spectrum of antimicrobial activity. It is effective against vegetative bacteria, fungi, bacterial and fungal spores and viruses, Instruments, lenses instruments, respiratory therapy equipment's and other special equipment's.

Gaseous agents

Certain types of medical devices are made from the material that can be damaged by heat and must be available in the sterile condition. Examples are plastic syringes, blood transfusion apparatus, and catheterization equipment. The same is true for routinely used laboratory ware, such as plastic pipettes, Petri dishes and other equipment that is packaged and sterilized ready for use. The main agents currently used for gaseous sterilization are ethylene oxide, β-propiolactone and formaldehyde.

Formaldehyde as a gaseous agent is already discussed under section aldehydes.

Ethylene oxides

Ethylene oxide is a relatively simple organic compound. It is liquid at temperatures below 10.8°C and above this temperature it vaporizes rapidly. Vapors of this compound are highly flammable even at low concentration in air. This feature can be overcome by preparing mixtures of ethylene oxide in carbon dioxide or freon. The carbon dioxide-ethylene oxide and Freon-ethylene oxide are nonflammable. The most desirable feature of ethylene oxide is its power to penetrate. It will pass through and sterilize the large packages of materials, bundles of cloth and even certain plastics. The concentration, temperature and humidity of ethylene oxide are critical factors which determine the time required to achieve sterilization.

Mode of action

The actual mode of action of this compound is believed to be alkylation reaction with organic compounds such as enzymes and other proteins. Alkylation consists in the replacement of an active hydrogen atom in an organic compound. In this reaction the ring in the ethylene oxide molecule splits and attaches itself where the hydrogen was originally there. This reaction would inactivate the enzyme with a sulfhydryl group.

Practical application

1. It is an effective sterilizing agent for heat and moisture sensitive materials.
2. It is used for disinfection of spices, biological preparations, soil, plastics, certain medical preparations and contaminated laboratory equipment.
3. It has been used in the space program by both the Americans and Russians for decontaminating spacecraft components.
4. It is used for its broad spectrum of activity against micro-organisms including spores, and also used as sterilizing agent because of its remarkable penetration power.

β-Propiolactone

It is the latest sterilizing agent. It has low vapor pressure and is a liquid at room temperature. It has boiling point of 160°C and it is non-flammable. It has less penetration power than ethylene oxide. It is generally used in the concentration of 24 mg/liter of space at 25°C. It is disadvantageous in terms of cause irritation, blisters, burns on contact with skin and it is carcinogenic.

Mode of action

Mode of action of this compound is by alkylation which is as same as that of ethylene oxide.

Practical application

It is used for sterilization of operation theaters, laboratories and aseptic rooms, etc.

VIII. METHODS OF STERILIZATION

The methods of sterilization can be divided into three main groups:

A. Physical Methods

1. Dry heat sterilization
   a. Incineration (flaming)
   b. Hot air oven
2. Moist heat sterilization
   a. Steam under pressure (autoclave)
   b. Tyndallization
   c. Heating with a bactericide
   d. Pasteurization
   e. Sterilization of vaccines
   f. Sterilization by boiling water.
3. Desiccation
4. Osmotic pressure
5. Radiation sterilization
   a. Sterilization by ultraviolet light
   b. Sterilization by ionizing radiation

i. X-rays (Roentgen rays)
ii. Gamma rays
iii. Cathode rays (electron beam radiation)
iv. Microwaves

B. Chemical Methods

1. Gaseous sterilization
2. Sterilization by disinfectants

C. Mechanical Methods

a. Filtration

A. Physical Methods

1. Dry Heat Sterilization

All the microorganisms also the bacterial spores can be destroyed by heat. This is due to the oxidation of essential cell constituents. Dry heating is provided at 100°C to kill all the vegetative bacterial in 1 hour but it does not kill spores. According to the pharmacopoeia, sterilization by dry heat is affected by heating at a temperature of 160°C for 2 hrs.

a. Incineration (Flaming)

Flaming is the simplest method of dry heat sterilization. In this method, the material to be sterilized is kept in the hot part of Bunsen burners flame for a few seconds and the process is repeated several times. Destruction of microorganisms by burning is practiced routinely in the laboratory, e.g. in the laboratory when the transfer needle is introduced into the flame of the Bunsen burner. Special precautions need to be taken to ensure that the exhaust fumes do not carry particulate matter containing viable microorganisms into the atmosphere.

Application

1. This method is generally used for those articles which are to be used immediately, e.g. forceps, needles, knives, blades, scalpels, metal spatulas, the mouth of culture tubes and bottles, and platinum loops.
2. It is also used for the destruction of carcasses, infected laboratory animals and other infected materials to be disposed off.

Disadvantage

This method is not reliable for sterilizing greasy or oily materials.

b. Hot air sterilization (hot air oven)

It is used for the sterilization of pharmaceutical products and other materials. Hot air oven is a double walled chamber made up of steel. Insulation materials such as glass fibers or asbestos are filled between the two walls of the oven to avoid heat loss. The door is also doubled walled which is having asbestos gasket on its inner side. Two or three perforated shelves are fixed inside the oven to place the material for sterilization. The electric fan is also fitted to ensure the uniform circulation of hot air in the oven to maintain the required temperature on all the shelves. The substance or articles to be heated are fitted on the bottom of the oven and it is thermostatically controlled. To note down the temperature inside the oven, a thermometer is fitted in the oven (Fig. 3.7). The materials to be sterilized are placed on the perforated shelves of the oven.

The precautions to be taken during placing the material for sterilizations are:

1. The articles and substances which are to be sterilized should not be placed at the floor of the oven because it may receive direct heat and becomes much hotter.
2. Glass apparatus must be wrapped with clean cloth or filter paper and containers must be plugged with non-absorbent cotton wool.
3. The oven should not be overloaded with the materials used for sterilization.
4. There should be sufficient space in between the articles, so that there is uniform distribution of heat.

The contents are heated in the oven for two hours at 160°C. The articles are allowed to remain there in the oven, till the temperature comes down to 40°C. Sterilized material is then removed from the oven

Advantages of dry heat sterilization

1. It is most widely used method for the substances which may get destroyed with moist heat sterilization or with moisture.

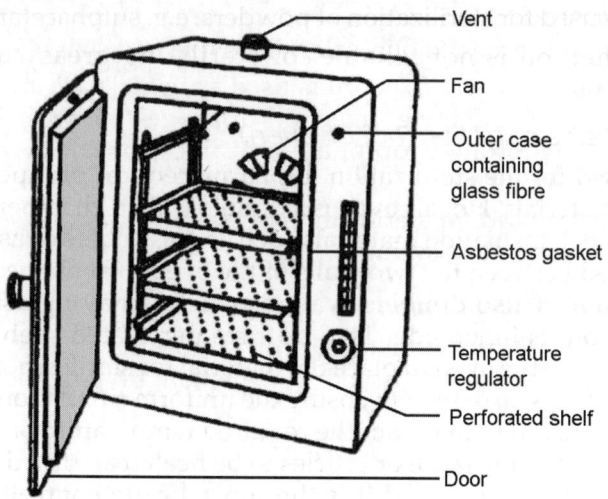

Vent

Fan

Outer case
containing
glass fibre

Asbestos gasket

Temperature
regulator

Perforated shelf

Door

Fig. 3.7: Hot air oven

2. The method is used mainly for the sterilization of assembled equipment's such as all glass syringes, flasks, test tubes, pipettes, etc.

3. It is not much damaging for the materials like glass and metal equipment as moist heat.

Disadvantages of dry heat sterilization

1. It requires very long heating time, high temperature and long exposure time.

2. The method is not suitable for most of medicaments, rubber and plastic goods as the articles are in direct exposure to a very high temperature for a long time.

3. Preparations containing water, alcohol or other volatile substances cannot be sterilized by this method as the liquids may evaporate at high temperature.

4. It is not suitable for a surgical dressing because the natural moisture of the fibers is quickly vaporizes. This leads to deterioration and ultimately charring of material.

Application

1. It is mainly used for sterilization of glass wares such as pestle and mortar, petridishes, flasks, pipettes, bottles, test tubes, etc.

2. It is used for sterilization of powders, e.g. sulphacetamides, sulphadiazines, kaolin, talc, zinc oxide and starch.
3. Injections where fixed oil is used as vehicle are sterilized by this method, e.g. injection of progesterone, injection of testosterone propionate and injection of oestradiol dipropionate.
4. It is also used for sterilization of scalpels, scissors, spatula, blades and glass syringes.

2. Moist Heat Sterilization

The application of moist heat for inhibiting or destroying microorganisms is discussed by the method used to obtain the desired result.

a. Steam under pressure

Heat in the form of saturated steam under pressure is the most practical and dependable agent for sterilization. Steam under pressure provides temperatures above those obtainable by boiling. Moist heat sterilization is more effective than the dry heat method. It is due to the fact that steam has more penetration power than the dry heat and the thermal capacity of steam is more than the thermal capacity of dry heat.

In addition it has advantages of rapid heating, penetration and moisture in abundance which facilitates the coagulation of proteins. The method is very useful for the killing of bacterial spores. The moist steam penetrates the spores and capsules of bacteria rupture it and escaping protoplasm is coagulated. The laboratory apparatus designed to use steam under regulated pressure is called an autoclave.

Autoclave

Construction: Autoclave consists of a strong metallic chamber usually made of stainless steel. It has cover (lid) which is fitted with the steam vent, the pressure gauze and the safety valve. Rubber gasket is fitted on the inner side of the lid to make the autoclave air tight. The cover is closed with wing nuts and bolts (Fig. 3.8). The electrically heated element is fitted at the bottom which heats the water and converts it into steam. The perforated inner chamber is placed on the stand. The material to be sterilized is loosely packed into it.

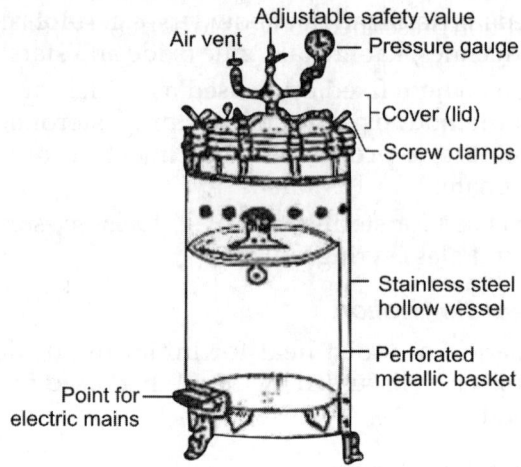

Fig. 3.8: Autoclave

Working

A sufficient quantity of water is poured into the chamber after removing the perforated chamber. The level of water is adjusted in such a way that it does not touch the bottom of the perforated chamber. The material is packed in the perforated chamber. The lid is then closed with wing nuts and bolts. The autoclave is switched on to heat the water. The vent is opened and safety valve is set at the required pressure. When steam starts coming out from the vent, it is continues for 5 minutes and then it is closed. It indicates that air has been removed.

The steam pressure starts rising and it comes to the desired pressure, i.e. 10 lbs/square inches with corresponding temperature 115°C or 15 lbs/square inch with corresponding temperature 121°C. Normally the following combinations of temperature and time are employed for sterilizing by heating in autoclave (Table 3.6).

Table 3.6: Time and temperature specification for autoclave	
Holding temperature (°C)	*Minimum holding time (minutes)*
115 to 118	30
121 to 124	15
126 to 129	10
134 to 138	5

The condition prescribed above is to be maintained throughout the load, during the holding period of sterilization. After the stated period, autoclave is switched off. Allow it to cool to about 40°C before opening the vent. When whole of the steam inside the autoclave is removed, the lid is opened and the sterilized material is taken out. In industry, large size autoclaves of both horizontal and vertical position are used. They are heated directly by introducing steam prepared in a centralized boiler.

Application

1. The autoclaving method is used for sterilization of surgical dressings and surgical instruments
2. The containers and closures are sterilized by autoclaving
3. It is used for the sterilization of most of official injections which can withstand the pressure of 15 lbs/square inches for 30 minutes.
4. Bulk solutions, glassware, surgical dressings, rubber gloves and surgical instruments can effectively sterilized by this method.

Advantages

1. Autoclaving method destroys microorganisms more efficiently because of high penetration power of steam under pressure than dry heat and hence the material is exposed to a lower temperature for a shorter period of time.
2. It is advantages for sterilization of a large number of official injections.
3. The equipment or parts of equipment, i.e. rubber and plastic (e.g. nylon and PVC) can withstand the temperature and the pressure required for sterilization.
4. A large quantity of material can be sterilized in one batch using a large sized autoclave.

Disadvantages

1. It is not suitable for sterilization of oils, fats, ointments, powders oily injections and other preparations through which steam cannot penetrate.

2. It is also unsuitable for the sterilization of injections and articles such as plastics and other materials which cannot withstand at 115–116°C for 30 minutes.

b. Tyndallization method

This method is a 'fractional sterilization' method. The method was official in B.P. 1932, for sterilization of medicaments which are unstable at 115°C but able to withstand low temperature heating. The method was used for sterilization of culture media.

Some microbiological media, solution of chemicals, and biological materials cannot be heated above 100°C without being damaged. If, they can withstand the temperature of free flowing steam (100°C), it is possible to sterilize them by Tyndallization. In this method, the solution which has to be sterilized is packed and sealed in its final container and heated at 80°C for 1 hour on each of three successive days with incubation periods in between.

The first heating destroys the vegetative cells but not the bacterial spores. These bacterial spores germinate into the vegetative forms in the interval between the first and the second heating and are killed in the second heating. Third heating provides a safeguard against any spores which may not germinate until the second interval.

The apparatus knows as the "Steam Arnold" is used for this technique. It is also possible to operate an autoclave with free flowing steam for this purpose. The method was deleted from the B.P. 1932 by the 4th Addendum (1941) and replaced by "Heating with a Bactericide".

c. Heating with a Bactericide

This is a special method of moist heat sterilization operates at 100°C. It is used for sterilizing aqueous solutions and suspensions that are destroyed by high temperatures of autoclaving. The suitable proportion of bactericide is added to the solutions to be sterilized. This solution with bactericide is distributed in final containers and sealed. The sealed containers are then heated at 100°C for 30 minutes in a steam sterilizer or water bath. This method is based on the fact that killing is done by heat as well as by bactericide; rather, the bactericides are more effective at high temperatures than at low temperatures.

The examples of most commonly used bactericides include benzalkonium chloride 0.01%, chlorocresol 0.2%, phenylmercuric acetate 0.002% and phenylmercuric nitrate 0.002%.

Disadvantages

1. The method should not be used for intravenous injections when a single dose of solution is more than 15 ml.
2. Similarly preparation meant for intrathecal and intracisternal injections should not be prepared by this method.

d. Pasteurization

Milk, cream and certain alcoholic beverages (beer and wine) are subjected to a controlled heat treatment called pasteurization. The method kills microorganisms of certain types but does not destroy all organisms. It is partial sterilization method which is used to make milk safe and also to improve its keeping properties. Pasteurized milk is not sterile milk. The process kills only 97 to 99% microorganism, but it does not kill bacterial spores. There are two methods used for pasteurization of milk they are as under:

1. Low temperature Holding (Holder) Method

In this method the milk is heated at 62.8°C for 30 minutes in a steam jacketed stainless steel tank containing agitators. This provides correct exposure throughout the milk and prevents skin formation.

Clean dry steam is blown to the spare above the liquid to prevent the formation of skin and foam. The method kills all types of bacteria including *Mycobacterium tuberculosis.*

2. High Temperature Short Time (Flash) Method

In this method, the milk is heated to 71.6°C for 15 seconds and quickly cooled. Here the milk is processed in special type of apparatus. The milk is placed in the narrow horizontal pipe and the large pipe will cover the narrow pipe which contains. The outer large pipe contains water.

The milk is heated by passing through narrow horizontal pipes inside large ones through which water passes in the opposite direction.

Advantages

1. The method is commonly used by most of firms because it is a less time consuming process.
2. It also needs less floor space and it is a continuous process.

e. Sterilization of vaccines

Vaccine is nothing but suspension of dead bacteria. The organisms are killed in such a manner that its antigenic power is preserved. Because the method used to kill the organisms depends on the stability of their antigens, because little or no immunity is produced if these are damaged.

The suspension of microorganism is prepared in the normal saline solution and then it is transferred into a sealed container. Sterilizations carried out by immersing the container in thermostatically controlled water bath at a temperature between 55° and 60°C for 1 hour. Strict aseptic precautions are observed to exclude any possibility of contamination. The vaccine is tested for sterility to confirm the proper sterilization of vaccine.

f. Sterilization by boiling water

This method uses the boiling water bath or electric boiling water sterilizer. It is useful for sterilizing the instrument like syringes, needles, knives, blades, scalpels, scissors and other surgical instruments.

They should be completely dipped in boiling water and should be boiled at least for 20 minutes. After sterilization the materials should be removed with forceps. The forceps are already sterilized by dipping the suitable disinfectant or by heating in flame.

3. Desiccation

Desiccation of the microbial cell causes a cessation of metabolic activity which then cause decline in the total viable population.

The time of survival of microorganisms after desiccation varies, depending on the following factors:

1. The kind of microorganism
2. The material in or on which the organisms are dried
3. The completeness of the drying process
4. The physical conditions to which the dried organisms are exposed, e.g. light, temperature and humidity

In this process of desiccation (lyophilization), the organisms are subjected to extreme dehydration in the frozen state and then they are sealed in a vacuum. In this condition, desiccated (lyophilized) cultures of microorganisms remain viable for many years.

Examples

1. Species of *gram-negative cocci* such as *Gonococci* and *Meningococci* are very sensitive to desiccation. They die in a matter of hours.
2. *Streptococci* are much more resistant; some of them survive weeks after being dried.
3. The *Tubercle bacillus* dried in sputum remains viable for even longer periods of time.
4. Dried spores of microorganisms are known to remain viable indefinitely.

4. Osmotic Pressure

When two solutions with the different concentration of solute are separated by a semi permeable membrane, water passes through the membrane, in the direction of higher concentration. This is to equalize the concentration of solute on the both sides of the membrane.

The solute concentration within microbial cells is approximately 0.95%. Thus if cells are exposed to solutions with higher solute concentration, water will be drawn out of the cell. The process is called 'plasmolysis'. The reverse process, that is passage of water from a low solute concentration into the cell, is termed 'plasmoptysis'. The pressure built up within the cell as a result of this water intake is termed 'osmotic pressure'. These phenomena can be observed more conveniently with animal cells because they do not have rigid cell walls. Plasmolysis results in dehydration of the cell and thus the metabolic processes are retarded partially or completely. The antimicrobial effect shown by this method is similar to that caused by desiccation. Because of the great rigidity of microbial cell walls (except protozoa), the cell wall structure does not exhibit the distortions because of plasmolysis or plasmoptysis. The changes in the cytoplasmic membrane and shrinkage of the protoplast from the cell wall can be observed during plasmolysis.

5. Radiation Sterilization

Energy transmitted through space in a variety of forms is called 'radiation'.

Radiation energies

The energies of electromagnetic and particulate radiations are expressed by quanta or photons and the unit is electron-volts (eV). The quantum energy of the most effective UV light for sterilization purposes is about 5 eV. The quanta of gamma rays emitted from 60 Co have energies of 1.33 and 1.17 MeV while the energy for the high velocity electrons is 4 MeV. By comparing these energies the low ionizing power of ultraviolet light.

a. Sterilization by ultraviolet light

The ultraviolet portion of the spectrum includes all radiations from 150 to 3900 Å. Direct sunlight can destroy microorganisms on account of its ultraviolet rays of long wavelength. The sun emits both ultraviolet rays of longer wavelength as well as shorter wavelength. The ultraviolet rays of shorter wave length are filtered out and absorbed by the earth's atmosphere (ozone, clouds and smoke). The antimicrobial activity of UV light depends on its wavelength (Table 3.7). This activity is maximum at 265 nm wavelength.

Ultraviolet light can be generated by passing a low current at high voltage through mercury vapor in an evacuated glass tube. Many lamps are available which emit a high concentration of ultraviolet light in the most effective region 260 to 270 nm. Germicidal lamps, which emit UV radiations, are widely used to reduce microbial populations.

The wavelength of 265 nm and adjacent wavelengths are strongly absorbed by nucleoproteins and disruption of these

Table 3.7: Antimicrobial activity of UV light at various wavelengths

Wavelength (nm)	Antimicrobial activity (%)
220	25
253.7	97
265	100
30	10
320	0.4

vital molecules causes fatal damage to microorganisms. Quartz and Vycor glass tubes are used for making the UV tubes as ordinary glass absorbs the antimicrobial wavelengths of UV due to presence of impurities like ferric ion, sulphur iodine and titanium.

Mode of action

UV light is absorbed by many cellular materials but most significantly it is absorbed by the nucleic acids, where it does the most damage. The absorption and subsequent reactions are mainly in the pyrimidines of the nucleic acid. These pyrimidines can be modified into pyrimidine dimer. Unless these dimmers are removed by specific intracellular enzymes, DNA replication can be inhibited and mutations can result.

Applications

1. They are used for sterilization of air to prevent cross infection in hospitals
2. They are also used for sterilization and maintenance of aseptic area in the pharmaceutical industry.
3. They are used for sterilization of thermolabile substances before packing
4. They are also used for sterilization of surface of working tables and rooms where aseptic technique is to be performed.

Disadvantages

1. Ultra violet rays have a low penetration power, so it is not applicable to sterilization of packed pharmaceuticals.
2. If the relative humidity is high, UV rays are less effective against organisms in the atmosphere or on the surfaces.
3. These types of radiations can be partially screened by dust or grease on the UV lamp. So regular cleaning or lamp is necessary.
4. Ultra violet light is harmful for worker. The eyes and skin should be protected from direct ultraviolet rays.

b. Sterilization by Ionizing Radiation

The ionizing radiations are:

  i. X-rays

ii. Gamma rays

iii. Cathode rays (electron beam radiation)

These are lethal to bacterial cell and destroy the nuclei of the cell. The material to be sterilized is packed in the final container and then exposed to ionizing radiation. Ionizing radiations are much more efficient as a sterilizing agent than ultraviolet rays.

i. X-rays: They are lethal to microorganisms and higher forms of life. Unlike ultraviolet radiations they have efficient energy and penetration ability. But they are impractical for purposes of controlling microbial populations because of two reasons.

1. They are very expensive to produce in quantity
2. They are difficult to utilize efficiently, since the radiations are given off in all directions from their point of origin.

They are widely employed experimentally to produce microbial mutants.

ii. Gamma rays: They are obtained from radio-active isotopes of cobalt 60. When the unstable atoms of this isotope disintegrate, they emit two gamma rays in succession. They can also be produced from radio-isotonic source such as ^{137}Cs or of electrons energized by a suitable electron accelerator.

As a result of research with atomic energy, large quantities of radioisotopes have become available as by-products of atomic fission. The radiant-energy particle makes a 'direct hit' on some essential substance such as DNA within the bacterial cell, causing ionization which results in the death of the cells.

iii. Cathode rays (electron beam radiation): When a high-voltage potential is established between a cathode and an anode in an evacuated tube, the cathode emits the beams of electrons, called 'cathode rays' or 'electron beams'.

Special types of equipment have been designed which produce electrons of very high intensities, and these electrons are accelerated to extremely high velocities. These electrons are microbicidal and also having other effects on biological and non-biological materials. The material by this process can be sterilized in its final package and at room temperature.

Application of sterilization by ionizing radiation

1. It is mainly used for sterilization of plastic syringes, hypodermic needles, scalpels, surgical blades and adhesive dressings.
2. It is used for sterilization of thermolabile medicaments.
3. It is also used for sterilization of bone and tissue transplant, plastic tubing catheters and sutures.

Advantages of sterilization by ionizing radiation

1. Gamma rays have a high penetration power. So materials can be sterilized after filling them in the final container.
2. Aseptic precautions are not required.
3. The temperature rise is negligible.
4. Some bacterial and viral vaccines can be sterilized without any loss of their antigenic power.
5. It is reliable method and the process can be accurately controlled.
6. The process is continuous because exposure time is very short so, the large quantity of material can be sterilized.

Disadvantages of sterilization by ionizing radiation

1. The plant used for this method is very costly.
2. The process cannot be stopped once it is started because the radiation cannot be switched off.
3. It produces the undesirable changes in many medicaments such as, colour, solubility and texture of product.
4. The radiations are harmful to workers.

B. Chemical Methods

Refer topic VII 'The major group of chemical used as disinfectant'.

C. Mechanical Method

Filtration

Sterilization by filtration is one of the oldest methods of sterilization used in pharmaceutical industries mainly for small scale filtration operations. In this method, the solutions which are to be sterilized are passed through bacteria proof filters. Examples of such bacterial proof filters include

Berkefeld, Pasteur-Chamberland, Seitz and Millipore filters. This method is very useful for thermolabile solutions and also for other solutions.

By this method, the microorganisms can be physically removed by adsorption on the filter medium or by a sieving mechanism. The bacteria are entrapped in the pores of the filter and then thus they are removed from the solution. Since, the filtration through these pores is very slow, vacuum and/or pressure are employed to enhance the filtration.

Practically, the filter, the accessories and the receiving vessels must be sterilized by suitable means and maintained sterile throughout the operation. This method requires, that aseptic conditions must be maintained. The apparatus should be thoroughly inspected before use if they are not cracked or breakage. This may render it unfit for sterilization purposes. After passing the solution through bacteria proof filters, the solution is distributed into sterile containers, under aseptic conditions. The containers are then sealed.

Although, all the processes, i.e. filtration, filling and sealing are done under aseptic conditions but still the microorganisms may enter into the solution from atmosphere or containers. So, sterility tests must be performed on the filled containers.

Three main stages are involved in the filtration process for the solution as under:

1. Passage of the solution to be sterilized through a previously sterilized filter-unit

2. Aseptic transference of the filtrate to sterile containers which are then sealed aseptically

3. Tests for sterility are carried out on the filtered product.

There are numbers of hazards in filtration sterilization and so bacteriostatic is usually included in the solution.

Advantages of sterilization by filtration

1. No heating is used so ideal for Thermolabile solutions

2. Removes all bacteria and fungi and often clarifies the solution

3. Useful for sterilization of large volume solutions

4. Useful for eye drops, as dropper bottles do not withstand the heating process well.

Disadvantages of sterilization by filtration

1. Aseptic technique required. This requires highly trained staff and sterile equipment and facilities
2. Sterility tests is required
3. Viruses, filterable form of bacteria and bacterial products such as toxins and pyrogens cannot be removed or destroyed
4. Filter may break down either suddenly or gradually in use
5. Filtration unit may leak and permit the entry of non-sterile air. Thus filter units should have as few joints as possible
6. Some filter yields fibers or alkali
7. Clogging can occur with prolonged filtration
8. Filtration cannot be used for sterilizing suspensions
9. Oxidation may occur on large filters and so the medicament must be stable in the solvent.

Types of filters

Various types of filters used for sterilizing the solutions by filtrations are

1. Seitz filter
2. Sintered glass filters
3. Berkefeld and Mandler filters
4. Pasteur-Chamberland filters
5. Millipore filters
6. Membrane filters

1. Seitz filter: Seitz filter was developed in Germany and marketed under the trade name Seitz.

Construction and working: They are usually round but sometimes they are square. These filters consist of two parts. The lower part is fitted with a perforated plate over which a compressed asbestos pad is placed. This acts as filtering media. The asbestos filter pads are made in several porosities for bacterial filtration. Upper part has a valve through which pressure can be applied. 2 parts, i.e. upper and lower are joined together by means of winged nuts. The solution to be filtered is filled in the apparatus, pressure is applied through the valve and filtered solution is collected at the bottom in the sterilized containers (Fig. 3.9).

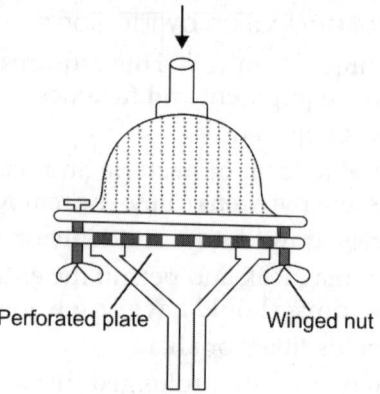

Fig. 3.9: Seitz filter

Advantages

1. As the pads are meant for single use, a new pad is to be used each time. This may minimize the risk of contaminating the filtrate.

2. The apparatus is very simple to use.

3. It is more suitable for viscous liquids than the filtration by ceramic or glass filters.

Disadvantages

1. Asbestos pads may shed loose fibers which makes the solutions unsuitable for injections.

2. The pads may adsorb sufficient amount of medicament which may result in the loss of volume specially when there is small quantity of the solution.

2. Sintered glass filters: It consists of ground glass particles which are fused together by heating to its sintering point. (Sintering point is that temperature at which the glass particles are used together to become solid, without melting). The fused particles have interstices between themselves which form a suitable system for filtration. They are prepared in the form of discs of suitable size and shape which are then sealed by heat into a Pyrex glass funnel, having the shape of Buchner funnel. This funnel is known as sintered glass funnels (Fig. 3.10). It is made in several porosities.

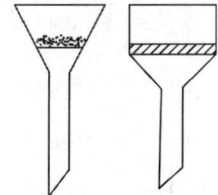

Fig. 3.10: Sintered glass filter

For bacterial filtration grade having the maximum pore size of 2 μm is used. For clarification of solutions, filters with other porosities are used. This filters are very fragile, so must be handled carefully. After use they must be cleaned thoroughly. For cleaning they must be washed by suction with hot hydrochloric acid and then with distilled water, until the medium is free from the acid.

Advantages

1. They are useful for filtering of small as well as large volumes.
2. Very little amount of medicament may be absorbed.
3. Volume of filtrate retained in the medium is negligible.
4. If the filter is properly cleaned, nothing can enter into the filtrate therefore they are specifically used for the filtration of solutions to be injected.

Disadvantages

1. They are very costly.
2. The medium is not suitable for large volume filtration because for that large discs are required which is mechanically weak.

3. Berkefeld filters: They are test tube shaped filters and they are also called "Filter Candles" or "Ceramic Candles".

Construction

They are made up of unglazed porcelain or kieselguhr and are available in various porosity grades. They are hollow cylinder shaped mounted on metallic joints. One end of candle is closed. The other end is fitted with a narrow opening which is attached to a vacuum pump when it is in use (Fig. 3.11). These

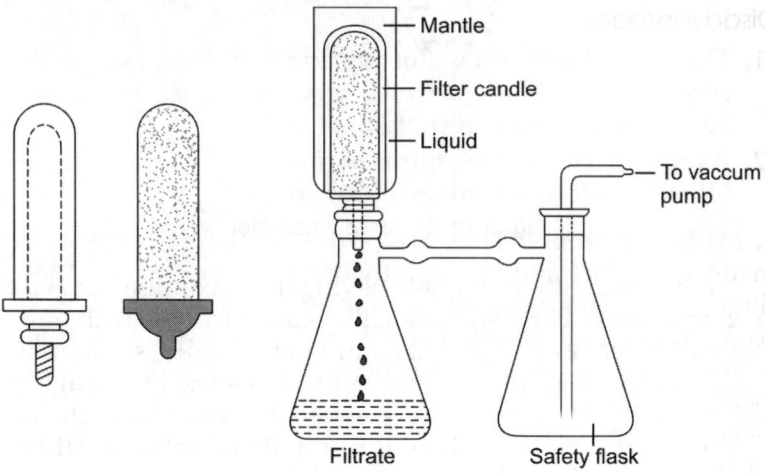

Fig. 3.11: Berkefeld filter

candles can be sterilized by moist heat sterilization at 121°C for 20 minutes.

Working

For filtration, the candle is placed in the solution to be sterilized. The narrow opening is attached to the vacuum pump. When the vacuum is applied and pressure inside the candle is decrease, the solution is pressurized to move inside the candle and this solution is collected in large size sterilized containers. The solution so filtered is distributed in final containers which are sealed immediately. The whole process of filtration is carried out under strict aseptic conditions. By the repeated use of filtration candles, they may get clogged and they can be easily cleaned by scrubbing the outer surface of the filter with the help of brush and by passing the water under pressure from inside to outside direction which will remove the entangled particles from the interstices.

Advantages

1. Thermolabile solutions can be sterilized without undergoing any changes
2. All the microorganisms, i.e. living as well as dead are removed.

Disadvantages

1. The main disadvantage of this kind of filters is that the pores may get blocked which requires thorough cleaning before the process is repeated.
2. As compared to other filtration medias these candles are little difficult to fit into the filtration units.

4. Millipore filters: They are porous structures which are made up of pure and biologically inert cellulose esters. These filters possess high degree of uniform pore size, high flow of solution and high thermal stability. They do not absorb the solution and are resistant to chemicals. Millipore filters are available in pore size raging from a high of 8 μ to a low of 0.01 μ. Generally a grade with pore size of 0.22 ± 0.02 μ is used for bacterial filtration.

Advantages

1. Among the various bacterial filters available, the Millipore filters are the most suitable and effective method.
2. Small volumes and large volumes of solutions can be filtered easily.

5. Membrane filters: Membrane filters have become very common among ultrafiltration methods. This is because the membranes used have been refined to a great extent. These filters are made up of cellulose, polyvinyl chloride, nylon and other cellulose derivatives. They are very fine having a wide range of pore size from 8 μ down to 0.22 μ. Generally for bacterial filtration, membranes with pore size of 0.22 to 0.45 μ are recommended. When in use, these membranes are fixed in a funnel of desired size and shape as like sintered glass funnels.

Applications

1. Membrane filters are extensively used for filtration and sterilization of a large number of pharmaceutical preparations such as parenteral preparations, ophthalmic solutions, biological preparations, hormones and enzymes.
2. They are also suitable for use in hospitals and in industries.

Advantages

1. Process of filtration is quite rapid.

2. Adsorption of medicament is negligible and only bacteria are removed by sieving because membranes used are very thin.

3. A few discs are used for every new operation.

4. They do not liberate particles or chemical substances to the filtrate.

Disadvantages

1. Fine pores may get blocked easily for which a prefilter may be used to remove colloidal matter.

2. When they are dried, they are very brittle.

3. Chemically they are less resistant and are soluble in certain organic solvents, e.g. ketones and esters.

Mechanism involved in filtration sterilization

Mechanical sieving

The filters like membrane filters have pores whose diameter is less than the dimensions of the bacteria. Thus removal of bacteria from the solution is by a simple sieving mechanism. However, other mechanism of filtration may also play a part since, majority of pores in candle filter; sintered glass filter and Seitz filter are larger than the bacteria. Example, candle filters have a maximum pore size up to 2.5 µm and yet can retain *Serratia marcescens* types of bacteria whose dimensions is usually less than 1 µm.

Electrostatic attraction and repulsion or adsorption on the filter The filters which have been insulated with oil may not retain the organisms from the aqueous suspension of bacteria which are filtered. Since candle filter, sintered glass filter and Seitz filters are negatively charged and the charge on the bacterial surface is also negative then repulsion rather than attraction may prevent the bacteria entering the pores. However, the attraction between the filter and local positively charged basic groups on its surface is also important. Thus both, the attractive and repulsive forces may play a part in the filter efficiency.

Retention in irregular cellular structure

Liquid filtering through a depth filter does not pass a straight through pore. An organisms passing along a pore in a sintered or fibrous Seitz filter travels a tortuous path that has a very uneven surface. It has been estimated that there are about 2000 irregularities/cm of pore in an unglazed porcelain candle. Bacteria may be stopped by or trapped in these hazards. The thicker the filter, the greater will be the delay. Bacteria originally arrested on projections in the upper part of the filter becomes dislodges as filtration proceeds and after a series of further filtration they eventually appear in the filtrate.

Imbibitions of water

The cellulosic fibers in the fibrous pad like in case of Seitz filter, imbibes water from the aqueous solutions. This causes the pad matrix to swell and thus there is reduction in the size of the interstices which provides more efficient retention of bacteria. Strongly alcoholic solutions cause less swelling and therefore organisms may pass through.

Standardization and testing of filters

It is necessary to show that the filter will retain the organisms and the flow rate is satisfactory.

The retention ability can be tested by following two methods as under:

1. Indirect method: *Bubble pressure techniques*
2. Direct method: *Bacteriological techniques*

Bubble pressure techniques

The direct measurement of the pore sizes of the bacterial filter is not practicable, so, indirect method of measuring the 'bubble pressure' is employed. In this method, the candles are immersed in water (or other liquid) in case of candle filter or funnel is filled with the liquid in case of sintered glass filter. Then gradually an increasing air pressure is applied until the first bubble is seen at the filter/liquid interface. The results are reproducible and it is possible to distinguish between the filters with a pore size difference of 0.25 µm. Bubble pressure method is adopted by a British Standard for measurement of pore size (Fig. 3.12).

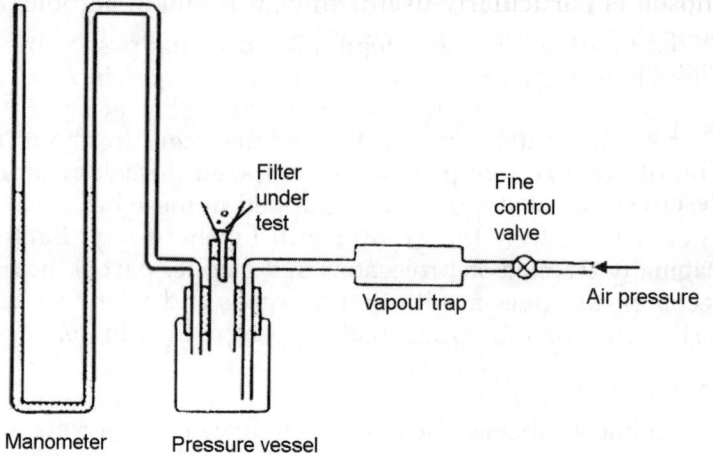

Fig. 3.12: Apparatus for determination of maximum pore size of bacteriological filter

The pressure when the first bubble is seen indicates the maximum pore size of filter which is then calculated from the equation:

$$D = \frac{30\gamma}{P}$$

Where,

D = Diameter of pore, in μs,

γ = Surface tension of the test liquid (dynes/cm)

P = Bubble pressure (mm Hg)

Bacteriological techniques

In this method, a diluted broth culture of *Serratia marcescens* is filtered through a previously sterilized filter and unit. A pressure difference across the filter of not less than 400 mmHg is employed. At least 50 ml of the filtrate is collected and incubated for five days and 25°C (the optimum temperature for growth of organism and pigment production), with addition of good chromogenic (pigment producing) strain. The appearance of pink color in the incubated broth instantly confirms the presence of *Serratia* and the failure of the filter.

Appearance of growth suggests contamination after passage through the filter or some leak in the unit. The organism chosen is particularly useful since it is small, aerobic, and nonpathogenic and grows vigorously to produce a red to pink pigment at 25°C.

IX. DIFFERENCE BETWEEN DISINFECTION AND STERILIZATION

The difference between disinfection and sterilization is described in Table 3.8.

Table 3.8: Difference between disinfection and sterilization

Sr. No.	Disinfection	Sterilization
1.	It is the process of removal of infection potential by destroying the microorganisms	It is the process of removing or destroying the all forms of microbial life
2.	The bacterial spores are not able to destroy by this method	The bacterial spores are also destroyed by this method
3.	It is done by using any of disinfecting agents	It is done by any of physical, chemical and mechanical methods
4.	It can be applied to the animate objects, e.g. antiseptics	It can be applied to an inanimate objects
5.	It is less time consuming	It is more time consuming
6.	High concentration of chemicals are used	Low concentration of chemicals are used
7.	Phenols, alcohols, heavy metals are the main disinfecting agents	Ethylene oxide, formaldehyde and ozone are main sterilizing agents

X. ASEPTIC TECHNIQUES

An aseptic technique is the one which is designed to prevent contamination of materials, instruments, utensils or containers during their handling.

Sources of contamination

The air

This carries mixed population of microorganisms and its density varies greatly with circumstances. In a dry period, the ground may become dusty and the dust can be swept up into the air by winds, which carries attached bacteria with it. Droplets expelled from the mouths of human beings and animals will also carry bacteria with them. From which the heavier drops may settle to the ground and the smaller droplets will be carried on the air will dry out and dispersed as solid specks. Mould spores are also in abundant because most of them are produced on aerial structure and dispersed by wind currents. Yeasts can be blown off the leaves of plants which often form their natural habitat.

The breath

During coughing and sneezing droplets can be ejected out from the mouth and can be propelled to a considerable distance. Apart from that it can also direct contaminate the articles being handled.

The skin

Although the sebaceous secretions exhibit some antibacterial activity, the skin usually has a great population of non-pathogens on them and also in the hair follicles and even sebaceous glands. In addition, touching the non-sterile objects with the hands also cause contamination by transient population. Pathogens and non-pathogens may be picked up when attending the toilet or blowing the nose.

The hair

Dust can easily settle on the hair and become enmeshed in it. If it is dry, shaking the head or simply disturbing the hair may detach considerable numbers of the dust particles.

Clothing

This also may carry a heavy load of dust particles unless freshly laundered which can easily be distributed and contaminate the articles.

Working surfaces

Dust will settle and collect on horizontal surfaces and to a lesser extent on vertical ones. This dust may contaminate the materials being handled.

Methods of minimizing the contamination level

Airborne contamination

This can be prevented by working in a room fitted with a fan drawing in air through a suitable filter. It can be also prevented by maintaining the slight positive pressure within the room so that the dust cannot be blown into the room from outside. The entrance porch fitted with doors at each end is usually provided to prevent the sudden inrush of air when entering or leaving the room. When designing the room, ledge (shelves) should be avoided on which the dust can be accumulated.

The breath

To avoid contamination from the breath, gauze masks can be worn, but these must fit closely to the face otherwise they may simply deflect the breath downwards on to the working area. The mask should be fine enough to provide complete filtration of droplets which will build up on the gauze or otherwise they will dry out and finally be discharged through the mask. The mask should therefore be frequently changed if working for long periods.

Contamination from skin

It is impossible to sterilize the skin without using the heroic measures which will be injurious to it. Careful washing will remove most of the transient flora and some of the micro-organisms. This also helps in cleaning away the dirt lodged under the nails. However, those embedded deeply in the crevices or ducts will not be removed even by the extensive scrubbing. Before operating any article the nails should be scrubbed and the hands and forearms washed thoroughly with detergent solution. The bactericide can be added to this.

The hands must not be allowed to touch any part of the apparatus or utensils which will come into contact with the sterile material being handled. It would be advised to add humectants to the washing water than a bactericide; alternatively a suitable cream could be applied.

Hair and clothing

The obvious course of action to prevent the detachment of the dust is to cover with freshly laundered material. Overalls or gowns should be worn over normal clothing and the sleeves should be rolled up above the elbow so that they do not pick up any foreign dirt from the unclean surfaces. A cotton cap should be worn on the head but if the hair is frequently washed and if an oily dressing is applied to it then there is no great risk of contamination. Long hair should be tied back for obvious reasons.

Working surfaces

Before operating, the surfaces of the working bench should be swabbed down with a bactericidal solution. Cetrimide solutions are useful for this because it has both the bactericidal and detergent activity. The surfaces of walls and ledges above the actual working surface must also be kept clean and the floor should be frequently swabbed to prevent the dust rising from it.

Apparatus and equipment

Glass vessels, containers and equipment though sterilized, some of their uncovered parts may come in contact with other non-sterile materials. They should be stored in dust-free cupboards and the exposed parts should be wiped down before use.

XI. PRECAUTIONS FOR HANDLING OF STERILIZATION EQUIPMENT

The main aim of aseptic technique is to prevent the contamination of materials, instruments, containers, glass wares, etc. during handling. The glass wares and containers should be thoroughly washed with detergent and water to remove the dirt and grease before sterilization. They are stored under aseptic conditions immediately after their sterilization. The aseptic work should be done in a special room which is made for this purpose. The arrangement is made in such a way that there is positive pressure in the aseptic room so that the dust particles may not settle on the surface of the apparatus.

The main sources of contamination are atmosphere, breath, the hands of workers, clothes, hair and working surfaces. To maintain sterility it is desirable to minimize the contamination which can be done as under:

1. By wearing sterilized gowns, face masks and gloves before entering into the aseptic room.

2. The hair should be properly covered with sterilized cap.
3. The hands should be thoroughly washed with soap and antiseptic solution before handling the sterilized equipment.
4. The working surface of the table or slab should be thoroughly cleaned with disinfectant before starting the aseptic work.
5. The sterilized equipment should be transferred from one place to another in a trolley or in a cart so that the aseptic room is not opened time and again.
6. The sterilized air should be introduced under pressure in the aseptic room to maintain sterility and positive pressure.

XII. EVALUATION OF DISINFECTANTS

Different tests are used to evaluate the bacteriostatic and bactericidal activity of disinfectant. A summary of the tests used is given in Table 3.9.

Table 3.9: List of evaluation test for disinfectants

Substance tested	Bacteriostatic tests	Bactericidal tests
Liquid disinfectants	Serial dilution in the fluid media	End-point or extinction time methods
	Serial dilution in solid media	Counting methods
	Cup-plate, fish-spine bead and filter paper methods	Nephelometric method
	Gradient-plate method	Use dilution method
	Ditch-plate technique	'In vivo' tests are applied
Semi-solid antibacterial formulations	Cup-plate method	Modified end-point or extinction time methods
Example, creams, ointments, pastes and gels	The ditch-plate technique	'In vivo' tests are applied, e.g. skin test
Solid disinfectants, disinfectant powders	Inhibition on seeded agar	Modified end-point or extinction time methods
Aerial disinfectants	Use of slit-sampler in test chamber	

A. Test for Liquid Disinfectant

Assessment of bacteriostatic activity

Serial dilution in fluid media (tube dilution test): In this method graded concentration of test disinfectant is incorporated into nutrient broth and inoculated with the test organisms. These tubes are incubated at 30° to 37°C for two to three days and then the results in the form of turbidity or colonies are observed. The results are recorded and the activity of the given disinfectant is compared as shown in Fig. 3.13.

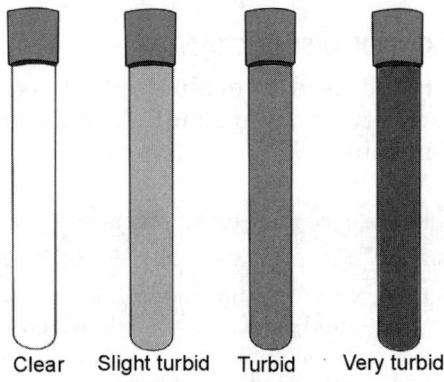

Clear   Slight turbid   Turbid   Very turbid

Fig. 3.13: Tube dilution test

The minimum concentration that prevents the detectable growth of microorganism (minimum inhibitory concentration— MIC) is taken as a measure of bacteriostatic activity. MIC varies with the different factors such as inoculums size, medium used and incubation conditions. These factors should be taken into consideration with each MIC obtained.

Serial dilution in solid media (agar plate method)

A suitable volume of double strength nutrient agar is diluted with the equal volume of bacteriostatic solution and this is then poured into sterilized petridish. When it is solidified, the lid is kept slightly raised and the surface is dried by incubating at 37°C for 1 hr. Drops of 24 hours broth culture of test organism are placed on dried surface and incubated for two or three days (Fig. 3.14).

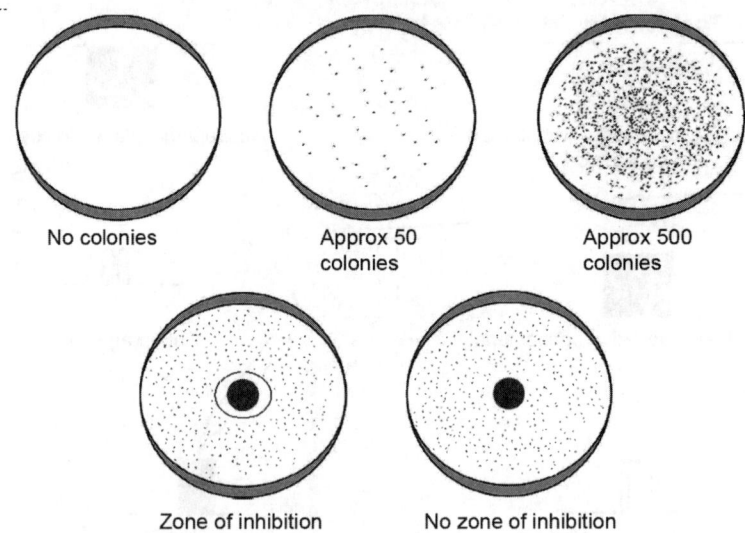

No colonies | Approx 50 colonies | Approx 500 colonies

Zone of inhibition | No zone of inhibition

Fig. 3.14: Serial dilution in solid media (agar plate method)

Up to 27 cultures can be tested on each plate if multipoint incubator is used. Plate with minimum concentration which inhibits or prevents growth is selected as MIC of disinfectants.

Advantages

1. The main uses of solutions are turbid bacteriostatic solution or a solution which gives turbidity with fluid nutrient media.
2. Solid media offer the advantage of economy, because a numbers of different organisms can be accommodating on single petridish.

Cup-plate, fish-spine bead and filter paper method

In these types of methods, the agar is melted, cooled suitably, inoculated with the test organism and then it is poured in to a sterile petridish. In the cup-plate method, when the inoculated agar is solidified, the holes about 8 mm of diameter are cut in the medium with the help of sterile cork borer.

In the fish-spine bead method, filter paper method and the cylinder method, the disinfectant is applied to the surface of the solidified, inoculated agar and in the cup-plate method it is placed directly in the holes (Figs 3.15 and 3.16).

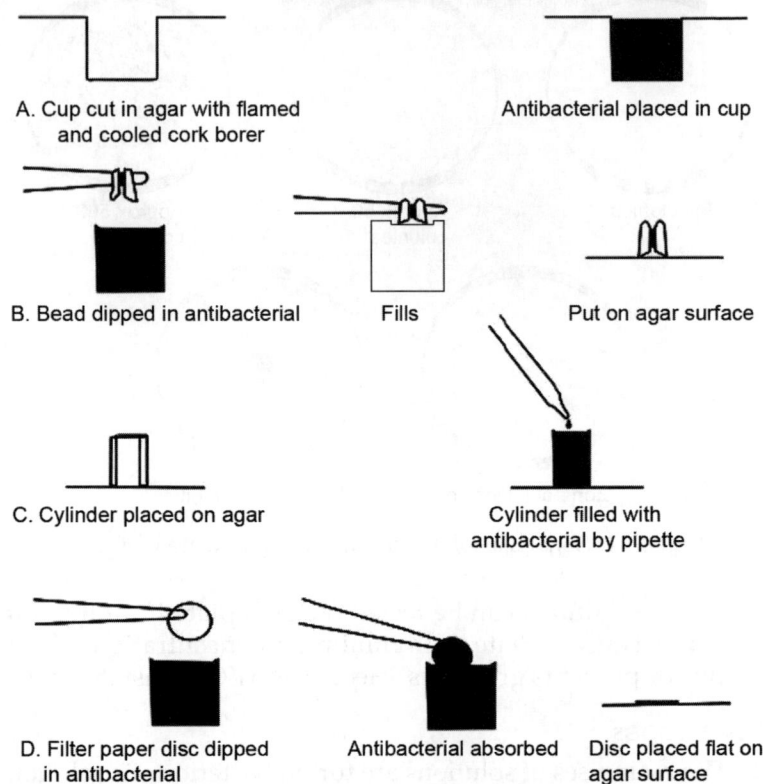

Fig. 3.15: Methods of applying antibacterial to inoculated agar: (A) Cup-plate method, (B) Fish-spine head method, (C) Cylinder method, (D) Filter paper method

In all cases, zones of inhibition may be observed; the diameter of the zones will give a rough indication of the relative activities of different disinfectant substance against the test organisms, or the effects of different concentrations of disinfectant substance.

Drawback

The method can give false indication because development of zone of inhibition is dependent upon ability of disinfectant substance to diffuse through the agar.

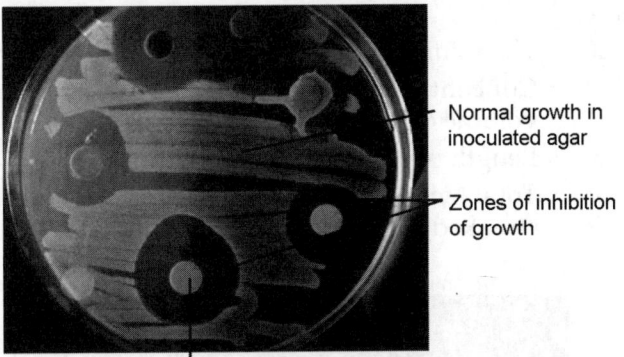

Normal growth in inoculated agar

Zones of inhibition of growth

Antimicrobial substance in cup (cup-plate method) or applied to agar surface (fish-spine bead, cylinder or impregnated filter paper disc)

Fig. 3.16: Assessment of bacteriostatic activity by cup-plate, fish-spine head and filter paper methods

The gradient-plate method

Two layers of agar are poured as shown in Fig. 3.17.

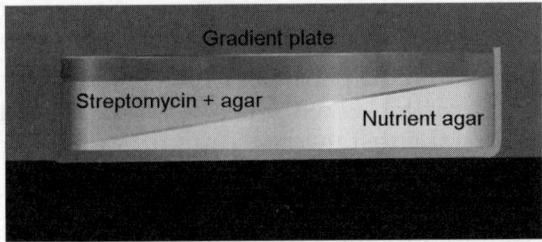

Gradient plate

Streptomycin + agar

Nutrient agar

Fig. 3.17: Assessment of bacteriostatic activity by gradient plate method

The plates are then incubated overnight which allows diffusion of the disinfectant substance.

The agar is streaked in the same line as the slope of the agar (i.e. along the concentration gradient) and re-incubated. Result analysis of gradient plate method is shown in Fig. 3.18.

An approximate MIC can be obtained from

$$MIC = C \times \frac{x}{y} \text{mg/ml}$$

Where,

MIC = The minimum inhibitory concentration

C = Concentration, in mg/ml, in total volume (i.e. volume of wedges A and B)

x = Length of growth, in cm

y = Total length of possible growth, in cm (i.e. length streaked)

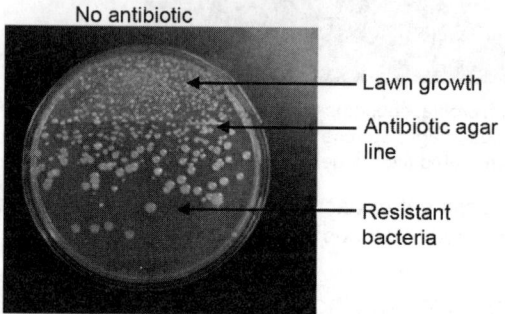

No antibiotic

— Lawn growth

— Antibiotic agar line

— Resistant bacteria

High antibiotic concentration

Fig. 3.18: Result analysis of gradient plate method

The ditch-plate technique

An agar is poured in the petridish which is allowed to solidify and a trough or ditch is cut out of the agar. A solution of the antimicrobial substance or a mixture of antimicrobial substance with agar is carefully run into the ditch so that ¾ is filled into it. A loopfull of each test organism is then streaked outward from the ditch on the agar surface of the petridish (Fig. 3.19).

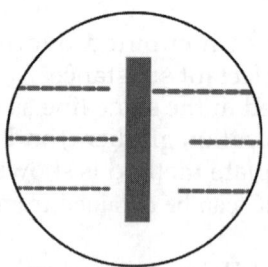

Fig. 3.19: Assessment of bacteriostatic activity by the ditch-plate technique

Six different test organisms show varying degrees of susceptibility to the antimicrobial in the ditch. The organism which is resistant to the antimicrobial agent will grow right up to the ditch whereas susceptible organisms will show the zone of inhibition adjacent to the ditch. The width of the zone of inhibition gives an indication of the relative activity of the various test organisms.

Assessment of bactericidal activity

End point or extinction time methods (phenol co-efficient test)

There are two types of extinction time or end point method.

A. Where, the extinction time is kept fixed and the concentration of disinfectant needed to kill the microbes in specified time will be estimated

These are referred to as phenol coefficient type of test and includes the following:

Phenol co-efficient test

1. Suspension test
   a. The Rideal Walker test
   b. The Chick-Martin test
   c. The United States Food and Drugs method
2. Surface film test
   a. Use dilution test
   b. Kelsey-Sykes method

Phenol Co-efficient test

This method is suitable for testing disinfectants which are miscible with water and which exert their antimicrobial action in a manner similar to that of phenol. The test organism employed in this method is a specific strain of either *Salmonella typhi* or *Staphylococcus aureus*. In this determination, the following factors are kept constant while estimating the activity.

1. The species or strain
2. The culture condition and number of microorganisms
3. The temperature and time of exposure
4. The sample size
5. The nature of the recovery medium
6. The time and temperature of incubation

Method

All the tubes (disinfectant + organisms and phenol + organisms) are placed in a 20°C water bath. These tubes are kept at the different specified conditions as per the different method and used for estimation of bactericidal activity. Descriptions of these methods are as follows

1. Suspension Test

Here, the suspension in aqueous medium is used for standard concentration of phenol and for a range of concentrations of the disinfectant under test.

a. The Rideal Walker test

Media : Standard Rideal Walker broth
Organisms : *Salmonella typhi*
pH of the medium : 7.3–7.5
Reaction temperature : $17.5 \pm 0.5°C$
Exposure time : 48–72 hours
Standard apparatus : Sterilized inoculating loop, glass wares, etc.

Method

To the numbers of dilutions of the disinfectant being tested, add 0.2 ml of 24 hr old test organism. At the same time, similarly, add the same amount of numbers of dilutions of phenol in other tubes. These subcultures of each reaction mixture are taken and transferred to broth after 2.5, 5, 7.5 and 10 minute (Table 3.10).

The broth tubes are then incubated at 37°C for 48 to 72 hours. Then they are examined for the presence or absence of growth.

Formula

Rideal Walker phenol co-efficient =

$$\frac{\text{Lowest concentration of disinfectant showing growth after 5 min but no growth after 7.5 min}}{\text{Lowest concentration of phenol showing growth after 5 min but no growth after 7.5 min}}$$

Table 3.10: Example of test analysis of Rideal Walker phenol co-efficient

Disinfectant	Dilution	Time (in min) for culture exposed to disinfectant			
		2.5	5	7.5	10
Test disinfectant	1 in 1000	+	–	–	–
	1 in 2000	+	+	–	–
	1 in 3000	+	+	+	–
	1 in 4000	+	+	+	+
Phenol	1 in 80	+	–	–	–
	1 in 100	+	+	–	–
	1 in 120	+	+	+	–
	1 in 140	+	+	+	+

(+) = growth; (–) = no growth

For example

$$\text{Rideal Walker phenol co-efficient} = \frac{2000}{100} = 20$$

It is not so that the idealized result shown in above example will be obtained in every occasion because

1. The reaction mixture transferred to the broth tube is random.
2. A few organisms shows abnormal resistance in the reaction mixture would also influence the result.

Some typical Rideal Walker co-efficient:

Phenol 1% in water (by definition)	1
Lysol	3–4
Roxenol	5–5.5
White fluid	10–11
Black fluid	14–15

b. The Chick-Martin test

It is more realistic method because the reaction takes place here is in the presence of a controlled amount of organic matter in the form of a standardized suspension of yeast cells.

Conditions

Conditions are very similar to the Rideal Walker test

Media	: Standard Rideal Walker Broth
Organisms	: *Salmonella typhi*
pH of the Medium	: 7.3–7.5
Reaction temperature	: 20 ± 0.5°C
Exposure time	: 30 minutes
Standard apparatus	: Sterilized inoculating loop, glasswares, etc.

Method

To the numbers of dilutions of the disinfectant being tested, add 0.2 ml of 24-hr old test organism. At the same time, similarly, add the same amount of numbers of dilutions of phenol in other tubes. These subcultures of each reaction mixture are taken and transferred to broth. The broth tubes are then incubated at 20°C for 30 minutes and duplicate samples are taken. Then they are examined for the presence or absence of growth. Example of test analysis of Chick-Martin phenol coefficient is shown in Table 3.11.

Formula

Chick-Martin phenol co-efficient =

$$\frac{\text{Mean of highest concentration of phenol showing growth in both the tube and lowest concentration of phenol preventing the growth}}{\text{Mean of highest concentration of test disinfectant showing growth in both the tube and lowest concentration of test disinfectant preventing the growth}}$$

For example

Chick-Martin phenol co-efficient

$$= \frac{1.8 + 1.45}{2} \div \frac{0.41 + 0.37}{2} = 4.15$$

c. The United States Food and Drugs method

Further types of phenol coefficient methods were developed in the United States of America which is also called the Food and Drugs Administration (FDA) method. This method uses the organism other than *Salmonella typhi* and includes the test for

Table 3.11: Example of test analysis of Chick-Martin phenol co-efficient

Phenol %	Tubes		Test disinfectant %	Tubes	
	1	2		1	2
2	–	–	0.47	–	–
1.8	–	–	0.41	–	–
1.62	+	–	0.37	+	+
1.45	+	+	0.33	+	+

(+) = growth; (–) = no growth

disinfectants used on the body, where, the *Staphylococcus aureus* is the test organism and the reaction mixture is kept at the temperature of 37°C.

Here, three types of recovery media are permitted

1. Normal nutrient broth which is for phenolic disinfectants
2. USP modified fluid thioglycollate medium, which neutralize the action of disinfectants containing the mercurials, other heavy metals or bactericides that act by oxidation.
3. Lecithin medium, which contains lecithin and the surface active agent, i.e. polysorbate 80, which neutralize quaternary ammonium compounds and chlorhexidine.

The medium that gives the lowest phenol coefficient for the test disinfectant is used.

Difference between phenol co-efficient tests

The difference between phenol co-efficient test is described in Table 3.12.

Advantages of phenol co-efficient test

1. They are inexpensive and can be performed quickly
2. They give reproducible results
3. They are valuable to eliminate useless products and supply standards for crude preparation

Disadvantages of phenol co-efficient test

1. Choice of test organisms: In the most tests only one organism is used, i.e. *Salmonella typhi*. Results for this organism gives only limited information on how the disinfectant will behave against other organism.

Table 3.12: Difference between phenol coefficient tests

Points of difference	Rideal Walker test	FDA test	Chick-Martin test
Medium pH	7.4	6.8	7.4
Volume of medium (ml)	5.0	10.0	10.0
Volume of reaction mixture (ml)	5.0	10.0	5.0
Diluent (for test disinfectant)	Water	Water	Yeast suspension
Reaction temperature (°C)	17/18	20	30
Test microorganisms	S. typhi	S. typhi	S. typhi
Sampling times (minutes)	2.5, 5, 7.5, 10	5,10,15	30
Calculation of phenol coefficient	Dilution test killing in 7.5 but not in 5 min. divided by the same for phenol	Dilution test killing in 10 min but not in 5 min divided by same for phenol	Mean of highest phenol concentration inhibiting and lowest permitting growth divided by same for test

2. Phenol coefficient tests compare the activity of bactericides at only one concentration with a fixed death time and reaction temperature.

3. Most phenol coefficient tests give no indication of the activity of disinfectants in the presence of organic matter.

4. These tests do not give any information related to tissue toxicity.

5. Sampling errors are large in this test.

6. This test do not give any indication of the effects of dilution on the activity of the disinfectant and are used to evaluate phenolic disinfectants only.

2. Surface Film Test

This method includes, the film of bacteria dried on the suitable surface. The surface includes cover slips, filter paper discs, and stainless steel plates or cylinders. The organisms are applied in the suspending agent that contains organic matter such as protein. After appropriate time interval the surface is incubated in a suitable medium. Mainly is it used in the determination of use dilutions test but occasionally used to calculate the phenol coefficient also.

In-use test

This method was described by *Kelsey and Maurer*. In this test, samples are taken from situations in which the disinfectant is used, e.g. liquid from mops, storage and rinsed liquids from urine bottles etc. One ml of the liquid is diluted with 9 ml of one quarter strength Ringer's solution (plus inactivators if necessary) and 10 drops are placed on the surface of an agar plate with a 50 dropper pipette. If not more than 5 out of the 10 drops show growth after 48 hour at 30° to 32°C, the disinfectant is considered to be adequate.

Assessment of systemic toxicity should be applied to wound disinfectants. The nature of the surface to be disinfected may also affect the choice of method of evaluation.

Kelsey-Sykes method

In this method, several test bacteria like *S. aureus*, *E. coli* and *Pseudomonas aeruginosa* are used. This test can be carried out in the clear or dirty conditions. In both the cases, the final concentration of the bacterial cells should be about 10^9/ml. the dilutions of the disinfectant are made in hard water

Procedure

Initially inoculate 3 ml of the disinfectant dilution with 1ml of bacterial suspension in broth, yeast or serum and shake gently. After some time (say at 8 min), collect the sample from above reaction mixture with a 50 dropper pipette. Transfer 1 drop to each of the 5 tubes of liquid recovery media or 5 drops to the surface of nutrient agar plate. After 2 min, to the bactericide/bacteria reaction mixture, prepared at the initial (time 0), add a second 1 ml of bacterial suspension.

Again at the same interval duration (after 8 min), collect the sample from the above reaction mixture with a 50 dropper pipette. Transfer 1 drop to each of the 5 tubes of liquid recovery media or 5 drops to the surface of nutrient agar plate.

(Reaction mixture now contains 2 ml of bacterial suspension). Again after 2 min, add third incremental addition of 1 ml of bacterial suspension to original bactericide/bacteria reaction mixture (a total of 3 ml is added).

Again after same interval (after 8 min), collect the sample from above reaction mixture with a 50 dropper pipette. Transfer 1 drop to each of the 5 tubes of liquid recovery media or 5 drops to the surface of nutrient agar plate. The samples taken at 8, 18 and 28 minutes are then incubated at 30° to 32°C and the number of tubes showing growth or the number of colonies/drop from the surface plate culture is recorded.

Interpretation of result

A disinfectant is satisfactory for use at the initial concentration if

a. No growth occurs in two or more of the five tubes of the 18 minutes samples, i.e. subcultures taken after second incremental addition of bacteria or

b. There are not more than 5 colonies from the 5 drops on the agar plate.

B. Test for Semi-solid Antibacterial Formulations

These include creams, ointment, pastes and gels. The base used for the formulation often affects the antibacterial activity of the disinfectant.

Assessment of bacteriostatic activity

Small proportion of formulation is placed on the surface of agar seeded with *S. aureus* and the zone of inhibition if any, measured. The technique was later modified by the incorporation of 10% horse serum in the agar to stimulate the conditions in a wound. The cup plate and ditch plate technique can also be applied.

Assessment of bactericidal activity

Modified phenol co-efficient tests can be used. Tests organisms must be well mixed with the semisolid formulation. Samples are taken at appropriate interval and placed in a broth which is capable of dispersing the base. Skin test should also be applied.

C. Test for Solid Disinfectants

In these formulations, the disinfectant compound is often mixed with an inert substance such as talc or kieselguhr to form a disinfectant powder. By dusting the powders on the inoculated plates, using the inert diluents as a control, the extent of inhibitory action can be ascertained.

British standard gives details of the determination of the Rideal Walker co-efficient for disinfectant powders. A weighed sample is shaken with distilled water at 18 to 30 min and the suspension used for Rideal Walker test.

D. Tests on Aerial Disinfectants

A closed room of approximately cubic dimensions and 1000 cu ft capacity should be used. The room must be initially free from the extraneous microorganism (by using UV light) and the temperature and humidity of the air is carefully controlled. Although in practice, such ideal conditions do not occur naturally. Fans should be incorporated to ensure uniform mixing of bacteria and bactericide.

Staphyllus albus is used as the test organism because it is the non clumping strain. Dispersion of the organisms into the air can be done with a collision inhaler. Samples of the air are taken at suitable interval with slit sampler. A bactericide achieving an 85% or more will kill in 4–6 min (RH 35–65%, temp 20°C) is considered satisfactory. Cyclopentanol 1-carboxylic acid has been suggested as a reference standard for air disinfection.

XIII. VALIDATION OF STERILIZATION METHODS AND EQUIPMENT

Definition of validation: Validation in the pharmaceutical and medical device industry is defined as the documented act of demonstrating that a procedure, process and activity will consistently lead to the expected results. It often includes the qualification of systems and equipment. It is requirement of good manufacturing practice and other regulatory requirements. Since the wide variety of procedures, processes and activities need to be validated.

Reason for validation: Validation is "establishing documented evidence that provides a high degree of assurance that the specific process will consistently produce a product meeting its pre-determined specification and quality attributes".

A properly designed system will provide a high degree of assurance that every step, process and change has been properly evaluated before its implementation. Testing a sample of a final product is not considered sufficient evidence that every product within a batch meets the required specification.

The validation process: The validation process consists of identifying and testing all aspects of a process that could affect the final test or product. Prior to testing of a process, the system must be properly qualified. It is essential for the sterile product to carryout strict control on them. Such controls must ensure the absence of viable microorganisms from the sterile product. These can be done by validating the process sterilization as well as by validating the products if it remains sterile for given duration of time. Validation of sterilization process can be achieved by the use of physical, chemical and biological indicators of the sterilization performance.

1. Physical Indicator

It is mainly used for validation of sterilization by physical method and mechanical method, i.e. validation of equipment and filters and radiation respectively.

a. Moist heat: Initially, the Master Process Record (MPR) is prepared as a part of validation procedure for particular moist heat equipment (e.g. autoclave) and for each sterilized product. This Master Process Record is then used as a reference record. Then for each next subsequent process of moist heat sterilization, the record is maintained for each Batch Process Record (BPR) obtained from a single thermocouple which is placed in a strategic part of each sterile product load.

The BPR is compared with MPR. The MPR should be checked at annual interval and whenever there is significant change occur in the BPR compared with MPR. Microprocessor controlled sterilization cycles are now a part of modern autoclaves. Pressure is measured by pressure gauges or through pressure transducers.

b. Dry heat: In the dry heat sterilization process, a temperature record chart is prepared for Master Process Record and each sterilization cycle for batch process is compared against master temperature record.

c. Radio sterilization: A plastic dosimeter is used for validation of radio sterilization. It gives an accurate measure of the radiation dose absorbed. It is considered to be the best technique among currently available technique for the radio sterilization process.

d. Gaseous sterilization: The gaseous sterilization is validated for elevated temperature, pressure rise, humidity, concentration of gas and leakage of gas. The elevated temperatures are validated for each sterilization cycle by temperature probes. Routine leak tests are performed to ensure gas tight seal. Gas concentration is measured by reference to the weight of gas used.

e. Filtration: Bubble point pressure test is a validation technique used for determining the pore size of filters. This test is also used to check the integrity of certain types of filter devices immediately after use. In this validation test, the filter is soaked in an appropriate fluid and pressure is applied to the filter. When the first bubble of air breaks away from the filter, the pressure difference occurs, this is equivalent to the maximum pore size of filter medium. When the air pressure is further increased slowly, there is general eruption of bubble over the entire surface and the pressure difference is equivalent to the mean pore size.

2. Chemical Indicators

Chemical validation of a sterilization process depends upon the ability of heat, steam, sterile gases and ionizing radiation of a variety of chemical substance to alter their chemical and physical characteristics.

a. Browne's tubes: Browne's tubes are the most commonly used chemical indicator for heat process. These are small sealed tubes containing reaction mixture and an indicator. When the substance is exposed to high temperature, reaction occurs and complete with producing change in color of indicator. As the temperature increases, four types of color change is being observed from red through yellow brown to green and to blue, the later color change is only being achieved after a specified time at the given temperature (Table 3.13).

Table 3.13: Types of Browne's tube

Browne's tube	Method of sterilization	Temperature (°C)	Color of indicator
Type I	Moist heat	126	Black spot
Type II	High vacuum moist heat	130 or more	Yellow spot
Type III	Dry heat	160	Green spot
Type IV	Dry heat infra-red	180	–

b. Witness tubes: Witness tubes consist of uniform diameter glass tube which contains a single crystalline substance of known melting point, e.g. sulphur (115°C), succinic anhydride (120 °C), benzoic acid (121°C), etc. A dye may be introduced into the tube to show more clearly that the temperature has been reached. The volume of the crystals and the diameter of the constriction of the tube is adjusted such that the time for transfer of the melt is the same as that is required for the sterilization oat the required temperature. Exposure time can be calculated by putting the crystals in the one end of an 'hour glass' tube.

c. Bowie-Dick test/heat sensitive tape: Heat sensitive tape is used quantitatively in the Bowie Dick test. This test is used to determine that if all the air has been removed from dressings and that if subsequent steam penetration has been even and rapid. The tape is suitably wrapped and placed at the centre of test pack. All the bars on the tape should change the colour which demonstrates the full penetration of the steam.

d. Royce sachet: The Royce sachet is used as a chemical indicator for ethylene oxide sterilization. This consists of a polythene sachet containing magnesium chloride, Hydrochloric acid and a bromophenol blue indicator. A given concentration time exposure to ethylene oxide results in the formation of ethylene chlorohydrins and a colour change from yellow to purple.

e. Chemical dosimeter: Chemical dosimeter is used for validating the radiation sterilization. It gives an accurate measure of the dose of radiation being absorbed. This is considered to be the best technique among currently available methods for controlling radiation sterilization. Qualitative indicators made of radiosensitive chemicals impregnated in plastic are also available. During radiation, the indicator changes the colour from yellow to red.

3. Biological Indicators

Biological indicators consist of a suitable organism to be deposited on a carrier and these organisms are distributed throughout the sterilizer load. The biological indicator validates the sterilization process directly by using microorganisms (Table 3.14). These indicators have ability to integrate all

Table 3.14: Biological indicators for different species of microorganisms

Sterilization process	Species
Autoclave at 121°C	Bacillus stearothermophilus
	Clostridium sporogenes
Dry heat at 160°C	Bacillus subtilis var. niger
Ethylene oxide at 600 mg/lit	Bacillus subtilis var. niger
Ionizing radiation	Bacillus pumilus
Membrane filter (0.45 μm pore size)	Serratia marcescens
Membrane filter (0.22 μm pore size)	Pseudomonas diminuta

sterilization parameter. The organism used for this validation technique should possess high and reproducible resistance to the sterilizing agent, should be genetically stable, should be readily characterizable and should be non-pathogenic. Some of the standardized parameters for accurate validation results are: the viability of organism, the storage condition before use and the incubation and culture condition after sterilization. At the end of sterilization process, the units/articles are recovered and cultured to determine the presence or absence of survivors. The microorganism used as biological indicators are usually resistance bacterial spores.

IMPORTANT STUDY QUESTIONS

1. Describe factors affecting disinfection process in brief. (Dec 2010, June 2011)
2. Enumerate methods for evaluation of disinfectants. Write a note on Rideal Walker coefficient (RWC). (Dec 2010, June 2011)

3. **Explain:** Thermal death point, Thermal death time, Iodophor, Bioburden, Bactericide. (Dec 2010)

4. Define 'sterilization'. Classify different methods for the same with mechanism of action. (Dec 2010, June 2011)

5. What is cold sterilization? Write note on fractional sterilization. (Dec 2010)

6. **Explain:** D-value, F-value, Z-value, Q10-value, Inactivation factor. (Dec 2010)

7. Describe biological indicators for monitoring sterilization processes. (Dec 2010)

8. Enlist methods for sterility testing. Discuss direct inoculation method. (Dec 2010)

9. Classify the disinfectants. Discuss the mechanism of action of any three. (June 2011)

10. How do you validate the bacteriological filters used for sterilization? (June 2011)

11. Write a note on an autoclave. (June 2011)

12. Draw a neat and labeled diagram of an autoclave. (Dec 2011)

13. Give advantages, disadvantages, applications and precautions to be observed in Hot Air Oven. (Dec 2011)

14. Write a note on gaseous sterilization. (June 2011)

15. Enumerate factors affecting growth of microbes. (Dec 2011)

16. Define disinfection. Enumerate five marketed disinfectants and give mechanism of action of each of them. (Dec 2011)

17. What is the effect of temperature and concentration on rate of disinfection? (Dec 2011)

18. Give merits and demerits of phenol coefficient. (Dec 2011)

19. How are the following items sterilized? (i) Ascorbic Acid injection (ii) Ethyl oleate (Give reasons for choosing the process) (Dec 2011)

20. How are bacterial filters evaluated? (Dec 2011)

21. Define the following terms: bactericide, sterilization, antiseptic, disinfectant, sanitizers.

22. Give ideal properties of standard disinfectants.

23. What is thermal resistance of microorganisms? Discuss the factors affecting it.

24. Discuss chemical disinfectant in detail.

25. Discuss sterilization by filtration.

26. Differentiate the disinfection and sterilization.

27. Discuss the evaluation of liquid disinfectant in brief.

28. Write about different phenol co-efficient test in brief.

29. What is validation? Discuss the physical and chemical indicator.

4

Analytical Microbiology

I. Analytical Microbiology
II. Microbial Counts
  A. Methods of Microbial Count
    1. Cell Count
      a. Total Count/Direct Method
      b. Viable Count/Indirect Method
    2. Cell Mass
      a. Direct Method
      b. Indirect Method
    3. Cell Activity
      i. Determination of Cell Count
        a. Total Count/Direct Method
        b. Viable Count/Indirect Method
      ii. Determination of Cell Mass
        a. Direct Method
        b. Indirect Method
      iii. Determination of Cell Activity
        Errors in Counting
III. Sterility Testing
    Sampling
    Culture Media
    Precautions Against the Contaminations
    Testing Procedures
    Control Test
    Inactivation of Antibacterial Substances
    Test for Sterility of Different Pharmaceutical Preparation as Per Indian Pharmacopoeia
IV. Microbiological Assay
  1. Microbiological Assay of Antibiotics
  2. Precision of Microbiological Assay
  3. Microbiological Assay of Vitamins
  4. Microbiological Assay of Amino Acids

I. ANALYTICAL MICROBIOLOGY

The term growth is commonly applied in microbiology refers to the magnitude of the total population. In the analytical microbiology the growth is determined. In this sense the growth can be determined by numerous techniques based on one or more of the following types of measurement:

1. **Cell count:** It is done directly by microscope or by using an electronic particle counter, or indirectly by a colony count.

2. **Cell mass:** It is done directly by weighing or by a measurement of cell nitrogen, or indirectly by turbidity.

3. **Cell activity:** It is done indirectly by relating the degree of biochemical activity to the size of the population.
   Other analytical techniques of analytical microbiology are:

   1. Sterility testing

   2. Microbial assay

Certain specific procedures will illustrate the application of each type of measurement.

II. MICROBIAL COUNTS

Growth in microbiology refers to the total population of microbes. This growth can be determined by numerous techniques based on the one or more of the following types of measurement.

A. Methods of Microbial Count

1. Cell Count

a. Total count/direct method
   i. Breed's method/direct microscopic count
   ii. Counting chamber method
   iii. Electronic enumeration of cell number
   iv. Proportional count method
   v. Wright's method
   vi. Coulter counters method/conductivity method
   vii. Packed cell volume

b. Viable count/indirect method

For aerobic type
  i. Plate count technique
  ii. Membrane filter count
  iii. Roll tube method

For Anaerobic type
  i. The Miller-Prickett tube
  ii. Ingram's method
  iii. Graduated pipette method

2. Cell Mass

a. Direct method
   i. Dry weight measurement
   ii. Measurement of cell nitrogen

b. Indirect method
   i. Turbidimetric method/photometric method
   ii. Nephelometric method
   iii. Colorimetric method

3. Cell Activity

Measurement of biochemical activity (indirect method)

i. Determination of cell count

a. Total count/direct method

The total number of organism in living or dead position, in a preparation is known as total count. In this, the number of cell is counted directly by an optical method or by electrical conductivity.

i. Breed's method/direct microscopic count

A microscope slide marked with a square of known area, e.g. $2 cm^2$, is used. A squared eyepiece micrometer is put into the eyepiece of a microscope. The area of the square and the number of squares in the area on the marked slide is determined.

The product in suspension form is diluted and a known small volume is spread carefully and evenly over the square on the slide. Then it is allowed to dry and then it is fixed and stained.

The number of organisms in about 40 squares selected at random is counted. From the size of the squares in the eyepiece, the area of film of suspension on the slide, and the volume of suspension on to the slide, the number of organisms in the original suspension can be calculated.

For example, if the area of the one eyepiece square is 0.0004 mm^2, the total number of squares in the total area of film is $400/0.0004 = 10^6$. If the mean number of organism per eyepiece square is 10, the total number in the film will be 10^7. Since this number was in 0.1 cm^3, the count of the original suspension is 10^8 per cm.

Advantages

1. Direct microscopic count can be made rapidly and simply with a minimum of equipment.
2. The morphology of bacteria can be observed as they are counted
3. Very dense suspension can be counted if they are diluted appropriately.

Disadvantage

1. If the suspension having less number of bacteria, e.g. at the beginning of the growth curve, cannot be counted accurately.

ii. Counting chamber method

This is a slide with a recessed area that is ruled in squares. A suitable dilution of the culture is made and a drop is placed on the recess and the slide is covered with plane cover slip, taking care not to trap air bubbles. The bacteria are allowed to settle and then viewed by dark ground or phase contrast illumination or they may be stained with crystal violet and examined by normal bright field illumination.

Usually two slides are made and the numbers of organisms in 4 groups of 16 small squares are counted, e.g. if the mean number of organism per square is assumed to be 10, the dilution of the original culture to get a suitable number per square is 100. The calculation is as follows:

Depth of recess $= 1/50$ mm

Slide of each square $= 1/20$ mm

Therefore volume above each square:

$$= 1/20 \times 1/20 \times 1/50 \text{ mm}^3$$

And if this contains 10 organisms, i.e. number of bacteria per mm^3

$$= 20 \times 20 \times 50 \times 10$$
$$= 2 \times 10^5$$

Consequently, the bacteria present in original culture can be counted.

Advantages

1. It is rapid method
2. Minimum equipment's and requirements are needed.
3. Morphology of microbes can also be studied.

Disadvantages

1. It is not possible to calculate the number of viable cells
2. Statistical errors may occur.

iii. Electronic enumeration of cell number

In this method, the electronic instrument, coulter counter can be used for direct enumeration of the cells in a suspension. It consists of the capillary tube. The diameter of this tube is so microscopic that it allows only one cell to pass at a time. The instrument can count thousands of cells in a few seconds

The bacterial suspension is placed inside the electronic particle counter, within which the bacteria are passed through a tiny orifice 10–30 μm in diameter. This orifice connects the two compartments of the counter which contain an electrically conductive solution. As, each bacterium passes through the orifice, the electrical resistance between the two compartments increases momentarily. This generates the electrical signal which is automatically counted.

Advantages

1. This method is rapid.
2. The instrument is capable of accurately counting thousands of cells in a few seconds

Disadvantages

1. It requires sophisticated electronic equipment's
2. Orifice tends to become clogged.
3. It does not give viable count because dead cells are also counted

iv. Proportional count method

The standard suspension of particles (plastic beads, number of particles/volume is known) is mixed with an equal amount of cell suspension. This mixed suspension is spread on the slide, fixed and stained. The particles and cells in the microscopic field are counted. An average count of the particles and the cell is taken from the number of fields.

For example, if an average count of 10 particles and 50 cells per field is obtained. Now, if the number of particles in 1 ml of standard suspension is 25,000. Then the number of cells/ml of suspension is $50/10 \times 25000 = 1250000$ cells/ml.

v. Wright's method

Equal volumes of the suspension and blood are intimately mixed and a film is made on the slide. This is dried, fixed and stained and the number of bacteria and red cells in about 40 fields are counted. The number of red blood cells in the sample may be assumed to be 5×10^6 per cm^3 or for more accurate work, can be counted in a haemocytometer (Fig. 4.1). Alternatively, a commercial standardized blood sample can be used.

As a ratio of blood cells to bacteria on the slide is known, the number of bacteria per cm^3 in the suspension can be found by

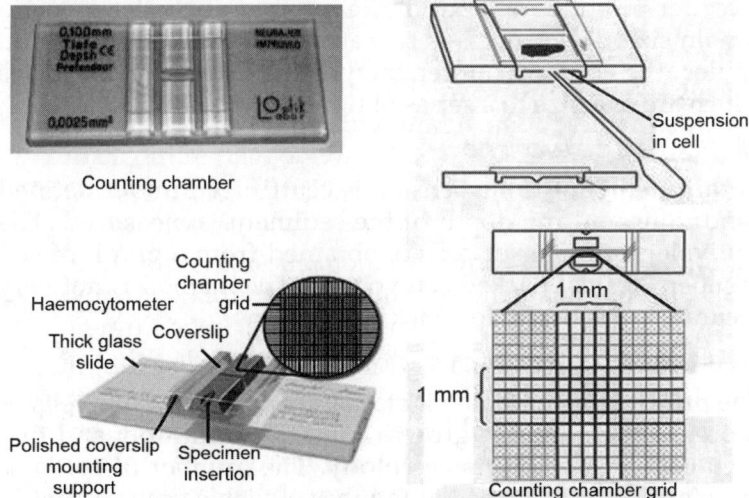

Fig. 4.1: Haemocytometer cell

proportionality. The sources of error in these methods are firstly, lack of homogeneity in the spread films (the Chi-square test can be used to detect this) and, secondly the small volumes used, particularly in the Breed method. At least three replicates should be done.

vi. Coulter counter method/conductivity method

Coulter counter method can be used for counting bacterial suspensions. In this method particles are suspended in an electrically conductive fluid and the particle size can be measured. The suspension flows through a suitable aperture with an immersed electrode on either side and the particle concentration is arranged so that only one particle travels through the aperture at a time.

As the particle passes through the aperture, some electrolyte is displaced and changes the resistance between the electrodes which causes a pulse in the voltage. The magnitude of the pulse will be proportional to the volume of the particle. This is a unique feature of the coulter counter, since it is the only method that measures a property having a direct relationship to the volume of the particle (Fig. 4.2).

The changes in voltage are amplified and impulses above a predetermined threshold value are counted, so that the recorder provides a count of the number of particles over a certain size. The process is repeated with different threshold values, the coulter counter carrying out counts of particles which are oversize to a series of pre-determined values.

vii. Packed cell volume

In this method, the suspension is centrifuged under defined conditions and the depth of the sediment is measured. The equivalent number of cells is obtained from a graph of cell numbers against packed cell volume. The method is not very accurate but is useful for thick suspensions.

b. Viable count/indirect method

The principle behind the viable count is that all viable cells or spores, under suitable growth conditions multiply and that each cell or spore forms a colony. The number of colonies therefore is the same as the number of viable cells present in the original samples.

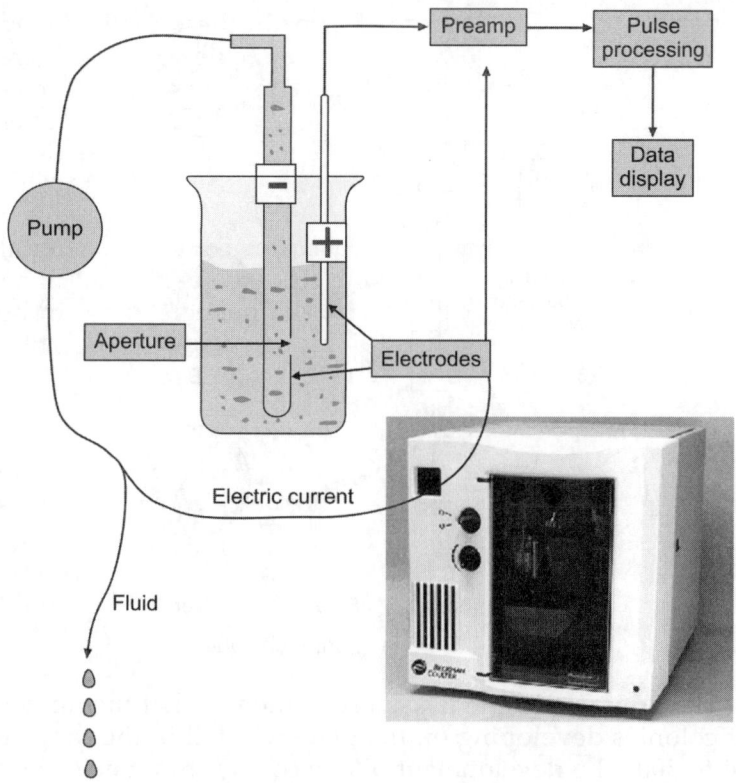

Fig. 4.2: Coulter counter

For aerobic type

i. Plate-count method: This method allows determination of the number of cells that will multiply under certain defined conditions.

A measured amount of the bacterial suspension is introduced into a Petri dish, after which the agar medium maintained in liquid form at 45°C is added and the both will be thoroughly mixed by rotating the plate (Fig. 4.3).

When the medium solidifies, the organisms are trapped in the gel. Each organism grows, reproducing itself until a visible mass of organisms-a-colony-develops, i.e. one organism gives rise to one colony. Hence, the colony count performed on the plate reveals the viable microbial population of the inoculums.

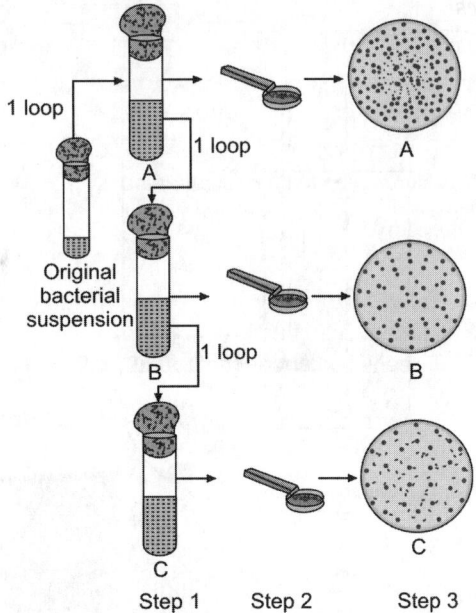

1 loop

A

1 loop

A

Original
bacterial
suspension

B

1 loop

B

C

C

Step 1   Step 2   Step 3

Fig. 4.3: Plate count technique

The original sample is usually diluted so that the number of colonies developing on the plate will fall in the range of 30 to 300. The development of one colony from one cell can occur when the bacterial suspension is homogeneous and no aggregates of cells are present, however, if the cells have a tendency to aggregate, e.g. *Cocci* in cluster, chains, or pairs, the resulting counts will be lower than the number of individual cells. For this reason the 'counts' are often reported as colony-forming units per milliliter rather than number of bacteria per milliliter.

Colonies are usually counted by illuminating them from below (dark field illumination) so that they are easily visible, and a large magnifying lens is often used.

Advantages

1. It is easy to perform and can be adapted to the measurement of populations of any magnitude.
2. It has the advantage of sensitivity, since very small numbers of organisms can be counted.

Disadvantages

1. The only bacteria that will be counted are those which can grow on the medium used and under the conditions of incubation provided.
2. Each viable organism that is capable of growing under the culture conditions provided many not necessarily give rise to one colony.

Uses

It is used routinely and with satisfactory results for the estimation of bacterial populations in milk, water, foods and many other materials.

ii. Membrane filter count: A very useful variation of the plate count method is based on the use of molecular or membrane filters. These filters have a known uniform porosity of predetermined size sufficiently small to trap microorganisms. This technique is particularly valuable in determining the number of bacteria in the large sample of air or water can be collected by filtering them through an assembly. The membrane, with its trapped bacteria, is then placed in a special plate containing a pad saturated with the appropriate medium.

Special media and dyes can be used to make it easier to detect certain types of organisms than with the conventional plate count. During incubation, the organisms grow into colonies which appear on the membrane surface.

iii. Roll tube method: Originally roll tubes are prepared by adding the dilution of organisms to a small volume of nutrient agar in a test tube, shaking to mix the contents and rotating horizontally, under cold water or in a block of ice. The medium is solidifies in form of thin film around the inside wall of test tube. After rolling, the bottle is incubated inverted for a time intermediate between those for pour and surface plates. The ideal number of organism is between 100 and 200 per bottle. The rubber stopper should be loosened during incubation to prevent lack of oxygen.

For anaerobic type

The solid media methods of counting described above can be used for anaerobes provided that the containers are incubated under anaerobic condition. Oxygen-free diluting fluids may be necessary. Other methods are also available for counting anaerobes

i. The Miller-Prickett tube: In this the organism is mixed with nutrient agar in a tube that is flattened oval in section and has a long narrow neck. The agar suspension fills the body of the tube and the neck is sealed with agar containing a reducing agent and an oxidation-reduction indicator. Colonies grow throughout the agar. They can be easily seen for counting because the tube is flat.

ii. Ingram's method: Here normal tubes or bottles are used. After introducing the suspension in agar, a thick sterile black rod is placed down the centre of the container and the medium solidifies around this. Because the agar layer is relatively thin and the organisms are viewed against a black background, counting is facilitated.

iii. Graduated pipette method: 9.9 ml of nutrient agar is mixed with 0.1 ml of culture, suck the agar by rubber bulb into the graduated pipette. Care is taken so that air bubbles do not enter the pipette—plug both side of pipette to create anaerobic condition incubate it for microbial count.

ii. Determination of Cell Mass

In this method, the weight or mass of the cells is estimated as an indicator of increased growth.

a. Direct method

i. Dry weight measurement: This is a simple and direct method of measuring the cell mass. The culture suspension is centrifuged and the pellet is repeatedly washed to remove all foreign particles. The residue is then dried and weighted. This method is mainly applicable in research investigation and for measuring the growth of molds.

ii. Determination of nitrogen content: The major constituent of cell material is protein and as the nitrogen is a characteristic part of proteins, one can measure a bacterial population or cell crop in terms of bacterial nitrogen. Bacteria average approximately 12% nitrogen on a dry-weight basis, although this can be viriated due to changes in cultural conditions or differences between species. To measure growth by this technique, first harvest the cells and wash them free of medium and then perform a quantitative chemical analysis for nitrogen.

Disadvantages

1. Bacterial nitrogen determinations are somewhat laborious and can be performed only on specimens free of all other sources of nitrogen.
2. This method is applicable only for concentrated populations.

b. Indirect method

This involves comparison with standard suspension and readings are taken with necked eye or by means of a photoelectric colorimeter or nephelometer.

i. Turbidimetric method/photometric method: Anyone who has seen the fog realizes that visibility is reduced in proportion to the density of the fog and the distance between the observer and the object that he/she looking at. This is because each droplet of water in the fog absorbs and scatters the light passing through it, and the more droplets in the light path, the less one can see.

Similarly, the bacteria in suspension absorb and scatter the light passing through them and appears turbid to the necked eye. A spectrophotometer (nephelometer) or colorimeter can be used for turbidimetric measurements of cell mass.

In this technique, the amount of light absorbed by the suspension is measured and then it is converted to numbers by reference to a calibration curves. The simplest instrument for this purpose is the colorimeter. It is simple and rapid method but, the method is relatively inefficient for low concentration of bacteria because they do not affect the response of the light detector, i.e. in the absence of particles it receives the full light. At the other end, the instrument is inaccurate when the suspension is too thick that organisms are obscured by others in the path of the light.

ii. Nephelometric method: The difference between this and the colorimetry method is that the instrument measures the light reflected by particles as the beam passes through the suspension.

In the absence of bacteria, no light reaches the detector. Nephelometers are more efficient than the colorimeters for suspension of low density but a point is rapidly reached where the refracted rays are further refracted by other particle and the result is no longer quantitative.

iii. Colorimetric method: In this method the amount of light absorbed by the suspension is measured and converted to numbers by reference to a calibration curve (Fig. 4.4). The simplest instrument for this purpose is the colorimeter but a more sophisticated alternative is the spectrophotometer in which the light of controlled wavelength is used.

The method is relatively inefficient for low concentrations of bacteria because these do not materially affect the response of the light detector which in the absence of particle is receiving full light. At the other end of the scale the instrument becomes inaccurate when the suspension is so thick that organisms are obscured by others in the path of the light.

iii. Determination of Cell Activity

Measurement of biochemical activity (indirect method)

This is an indirect method to determine the microbial growth. Measurement of a specific chemical change by metallic activities of microbes can be correlated with the microbial growth. Cell metabolic activity results into formation of any specific metabolite.

Example, lactic acid, H_2S, CO_2, enzymes, etc. The measurement of these products forms the principle of measurement of cell

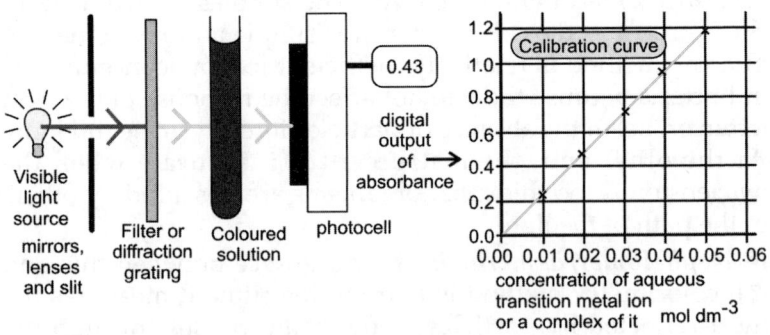

Fig. 4.4: A simplified diagram of colorimeter

activity. The amount of acid produced is proportional to the magnitude of cell suspension.

Errors in Counting

Counting errors are of following types:

a. Sampling errors

These occur because bacteria are not evenly distributed in the material under examination. There should be very little variation between samples from mobile liquids provided these are shaken well immediately before the samples are removed. With solid, semi-solid or viscous preparations (surgical dressings and ointments) it is more difficult to ensure that the sample represents the whole and portions should be selected in a random manner and be adequate in number and size.

b. Error of diluting and pipetting

Always considerable dilution is necessary to reduce the number of bacteria in a sample to a level at which counting is possible. At each stage error can occur while diluting and pipetting the samples.

c. Errors due to the culture medium

The medium used for counting should be accurately reproducible and uniform throughout; it should give maximum and concordant counts from time to time and batch to batch. Statistical tests are necessary to confirm that these requirements are satisfied.

d. Errors of counting colonies

Small colonies may be missed if a lens is not used. If the number of colonies is large, a hand tally or an electromagnetic counter is helpful. The counting of large numbers is also facilitated by dividing the container into small areas with waxed pencil lines and counting each separately.

e. Personal errors

These are related to the carefulness and technical ability of the worker. They can often be reduced, e.g. by holding a dropping pipette in a stand instead of the hand.

III. STERILITY TESTING

The tests for sterility are done by detecting the presence of viable forms of bacteria, fungi and yeast on pharmacopoeial preparations. The tests must be carried out under strict aseptic condition to avoid accidental contamination of product during the test and all the glass apparatus required for the test must be sterile.

Principle: Sterility tests are the tests which are based upon the principle that if the bacteria or fungi are placed in a medium which provides the nutritive material, moisture, the desired pH and are kept at a favorable temperature, the organisms will grow and their presence can be indicated by the turbidity in the originally clear medium.

For the following examples of some of the preparation, the compliance with the test is required.

1. Readymade injections
2. Solids for injections
3. Eye drops, eye ointment and eye lotion
4. Water for injection (free from pyrogens and metabolic products of microorganisms)
5. Human blood and blood products obtained from it.
6. All immunological preparation
7. Implants
8. Catgut
9. Absorbable haemostatic

There is one class of sterile products—injection sterilized by filtration—for which BP requires the test on every batch. Sterilization by filtration requires quite complicated aseptic technique and certain faults that can arise such as leak in some unit or defect in the filtering medium are not usually easily detected during process. Because the most therapeutic substances are very thermolabile, sterile products are generally obtained by filtration or aseptic technique. Every batch of final container must be tested for sterility and except in certain special circumstances issues are prohibited until tests are passed.

*The **special circumstances** are*

1. When preparation is required in emergency by medical practitioner and manufacturer has no filled container in stock provided that

    a. Bulk from which the containers are filled has been tested and has passed the test.

    b. Test on the samples from some of the filled containers are set up, examine daily and if contamination is detected, the practitioner is notified.

2. When the substance is so unstable that it losses the appreciable active if it is hold until completion of test. In this case bulk test is waived and only (b) is applied.

Example, liquid BCG vaccines are now replaced by freeze dried BCG vaccines which is more stable.

Limitation of sterility testing: In microbial sense, the sterility means the freedom from living microorganisms, and therefore, it is not possible to say that a batch of product is sterile until, entire content of every container in the batch has been tested. The test provides the optimum condition for growth and multiplication of all kind of microorganisms.

Unfortunately neither of these conditions can be satisfied because

1. In sterility testing article or preparation to be tested is either destroyed or made unstable. So, only part of the batch can be sampled.

2. Even great care is taken to provide a media and incubation condition satisfactory for all microorganisms, it is impossible to supply all variations necessary to ensure that every type and condition of contaminant can grow.

Consequently sterility testing can only show that the organism capable of growing in test media under the selected conditions are absent from the function of the batch that has been tested. Very low level of contamination can be detected on the basis of random sampling. Thus sterility testing does not give 100% assurance.

Sampling

1. Stages at which the samples should be taken: For the heat sterilized product, sample should be taken only from the final container. When processing involves aseptic technique, it is advisable to test final container as well as the bulk from which the final containers will be filled, e.g. The product sterilized by filtration can be contaminated during filtration process and during the filling process. Now, by performing bulk as well as final container tests, it is possible to examine that which stage is responsible for contamination.

2. Selection of the samples: Sample must be representative of whole of bulk material and the final container lot. For bulk, the material must be thoroughly mixed before the sample is taken. For final container, sample must be selected at random but,

a. *Heat:* when a load from a heat sterilization process is tested, sample should be collected from every shelf and every part of sterilized in which the less sterilizing condition is believe to exist.

b. *Filtration:* From aseptically processed preparation, samples must be taken throughout the filling operation.

c. *Radiation:* For product sterilized by a continuous process, such as radiation sterilization, samples are selected from total number of similar item subjected to uniform sterilization during an appropriate period, which the USP suggest should not exceed one day.

3. Sample size: Sample size depends on factors such as environmental condition, volume of the preparation per container, etc. IP recommended the minimum number of size samples to be tested for sterility. It is given in Table 4.1.

Culture Media

Culture media used for test may be prepared as described in IP. Culture media is required for aerobic and anaerobic bacteria and for fungi. The media used should comply with the tests, such as, sterility, nutritive properties, and effectiveness of media as per details given in IP.

1. Sensitivity

Sterility test media must initiate and maintain the vigorous growth of small number of:

a. Aerobic and anaerobic bacteria
b. The lower fungi, i.e. yeast and mould responsible for spoilage.

2. Types

Sterility test should detect bacteria, mould and yeast. Separate media are separately designed for aerobes, anaerobes and

Table 4.1: Number of size of samples to be tested for sterility

No. of item in batch	Minimum no. of item recommended to be tested
Parenteral preparation	
Not more than 100 containers	10% or 4 containers, whichever is greater
More than 100 but not more than 500 containers	10 containers
More than 500 container	2% or 20 containers whichever is less
For large volume parenteral	2% or 20 containers whichever is less
Ophthalmic and non-parenteral preparation	
Not more than 200 container	5% or 2 containers whichever is greater
More than 200 container	10 containers
Surgical dressings and devices	
Catgut, surgical sutures and other sterile medical device for use	2% or 5 packages whichever is greater up to 20 packages
Not more than 100 packages	10% or 4 packages whichever is greater
More than 100 but not more than 500 packages	10 packages
More than 500 packages	2% or 20 packages whichever is less
Bulk solids	
Less than 4 containers	Each container
4 container but not more than 50 container	20% or 4 containers whichever is greater
More than 50 containers	2% or 10 containers whichever is greater

lower fungi are preferred by some authority because they are most sensitive. Other experts believe that detection of as many organisms as possible, both type and number, it is most likely to be fulfilled by use of nonselective media such as broths that can support the growth of all types of microorganism Enough oxygen is present at the top, for the growth of strict aerobic microorganism. Gradient oxygen concentration for organisms with the intermediate requirement is present in between the media. Bottom condition is suitable for anaerobic microorganisms (Fig. 4.5).

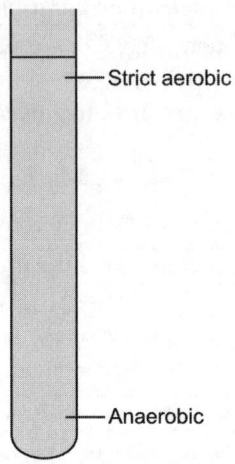

Strict aerobic

Anaerobic

Fig. 4.5: Growth of microorganism according to their types

1. For Detection of Aerobes

i. *Peptone broth:* It is meat extract broths containing peptone.

ii. *Glucose peptone broth:* It contains 0.5% dextrose which promotes the growth of many bacteria.

2. For Detection of Anaerobes

Cooked meat medium (Robertson Balloch heart media—RBHM): It is a suitable medium for growing anaerobes and also for the preservation of stock of anaerobic microorganisms.

i. Preparation of cooked meat

Fresh bovine heart	500 g
Water	500 ml
Sodium hydroxide (1 N)	1.5 ml

Mince the heart, place in the alkaline boiling water and simmer for 20 minutes to neutralize lactic acid present in the meat. While still hot press the minced meat in a cloth and dry partially by spreading it over cloth or filter paper.

ii. Preparation of pepto infusion broth

Liquid filtered from meat	500 ml
Peptone	2.5 gm
Sodium chloride	1.25 gm

Steam at 100°C for 20 minutes, add 1 ml pure HCl and filter. Bring the reaction of filtrate to 8.2 pH. Steam at 100°C for 30 minutes and adjust the reaction to pH 7.8.

iii. Preparation of complete medium

Place meat in one ounce narrow neck bottle to level of about one inch and cover it with about 10 ml of pepto infusion broth. Autoclave at 121 C for 20 minutes. The oxidation reduction potential of the medium is –0.2 volts and thus it gives anaerobic condition. Inoculation is introduced deep in the medium in contact with the meat.

Semi fluid meat medium (sloppy agar)

Liver broth—used for examination of food for anaerobes.

Although recommended for anaerobic microorganism, these medias contain sufficient oxygen in upper region to permit growth of aerobes. So, sometimes it is used as joint media.

3. For Detection of Aerobes and Anaerobes (Joint Medium)

i. Fluid thioglycollate medium (fluid merceptoacetic acid medium BP 93):

This medium is used with a clear fluid product (Table 4.2).

Dextrose and sodium thioglycollate act as a reducing sugar. Resazurin: As oxygen diffuses into media and spreads down from the top, oxygen deduction potential increases and indicator shows corresponding change in color from colorless to pink.

Procedure

- Mix the weighed quantity of the ingredients other than the thioglycollate and the resazurin in a mortar with thorough grinding.
- Stir in some heated distilled water.
- Transfer to a suitable container.

Table 4.2: Formula of fluid thioglycollate medium

Ingredients	Quantity	Function
L-Cystine	0.5 g	Encourage growth of certain *Clostridia* (source of amino acid)
Sodium chloride	2.5 g	Nutrient
Dextrose	5.5 g	Source of carbon
Granular agar (moisture less than 15% w/w)	0.75 g	Increase the viscosity and prevent the inward diffusion of oxygen into media
Yeast extract (water soluble)	5 g	Growth factor source
Pancreatic digest	15 g	Nitrogen source of casein
Sodium thioglycollate or thioglycollic acid	0.5/0.3 g	Reducing agent
Resazurin (0.1% fresh solution)	1 ml	Oxidation/reduction indicator
Distilled water	To 1000 ml	–

- Add the remainder of water and complete the solution by heating in a boiling water bath.
- Add sodium thioglycollate and then add 1 M sodium hydroxide if necessary, so that (after sterilization), the medium will have a pH of 7.1 ± 0.2.
- Reheat the solution but do not boil.
- Filter (if necessary) through moistened filter paper and add the resazurin solution.
- Distribute into suitable vessels that shows color change, indicative of oxygen uptake at the end of incubating period.
- Sterilize in an autoclave at 121°C for 20 minutes.
- Cool to 25°C and store at 20–30°C avoiding excess of light.

Suitability of formulated media

- Pink color is indicative of oxygen uptake.

The formula is suitable for detection of anaerobes if not more than upper 30% is colored (Fig. 4.6). The formula is suitable for detection of aerobes if the solution does not contain pink color at all. A medium that contains not more than upper

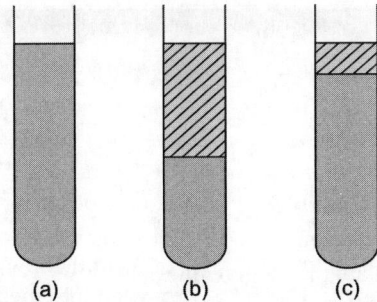

Fig. 4.6: (a) Completely reduced-suitable for anaerobes, (b) more than 305 colored—suitable as an anaerobic media, (c) not more than upper 1/10th region colored—used as joint media

1/10th region colored is more suitable as joint medium than a completely reduced medium because aerobic growth will be more quickly initiated. The reduced conditions may be restored by heating in a water bath until the pink color disappears; this treatment must not be repeated because frequent reheating gives rise to toxic degradation product.

ii. Alternatively thioglycollate media (Thioglycollate broth medium)

It is used with turbid or viscous preparation, e.g. semi-solids like creams and turbid preparation like suspensions. In comparison to fluid thioglycollate medium the agar is absent in thioglycollate broth medium (Table 4.3). It is used when the high viscosity of media prevents the satisfactory dispersal of certain test materials throughout the medium. Because it contains no agar to retard diffusion of oxygen, the medium must be heated not more than 4 hours before use.

Formula: Table 4.3 describes formula of thioglycollate broth medium.

iii. Corn steep liquor-sodium thioglycollate medium

It differs from the fluid thioglycollate medium (Table 4.4) in the following aspects:
- a. The nitrogen source is meat extract in this media instead of casein digest.
- b. The growth factor source is corn steep liquor instead or yeast extract.

Table 4.3: Formula of thioglycollate broth medium

Ingredients	Quantity
L-Cystine	0.5 g
Sodium chloride	2.5 g
Dextrose	5.5 g
Yeast extract (water soluble)	5 g
Pancreatic digest of casein	15 g
Sodium thioglycollate or thioglycollic acid	0.5/0.3 g
Resazurin (0.1% fresh solution)	1 ml
Distilled water	To 1000 ml

Table 4.4: Formula of corn steep liquor-sodium thioglycollate medium

Ingredients	Quantity
Sodium chloride	2.5 g
Dextrose	5.5 g
Corn steep liquor	5 g
Meat extract	15 g
Sodium thioglycollate or thioglycollic acid	0.5/0.3 g
Sodium hydrosulphite	0.5/0.3 g
Resazurin (0.1% fresh solution)	1 ml
Distilled water	To 1000 ml

c. It contains sodium hydrosulphite as an additional reducing agent.

d. There is no special supplement of L-cystine.

Formula: Table 4.4 describes formula of corn steep liquor-sodium thioglycollate medium.

iv. Semi-fluid hydrosulphite medium

The differences from fluid thioglycollate medium are

a. Sodium hydrosulphite replaces sodium thioglycollate as the main reducing agent.

b. Peptone replaces the casein digest.

c. The agar concentration is almost twice as large.

d. No L-cystine supplement.

Formula: Table 4.5 describes formula of semi-fluid hydrosulphite medium.

Table 4.5: Formula of semi-fluid hydrosulphite medium

Ingredients	Quantity
Sodium chloride	2.5 g
Dextrose	5.5 g
Granular agar (moisture less than 15% w/w)	1.5 g
Yeast extract (water soluble)	5 g
Peptone	15 g
Sodium hydrosulphite	0.5/0.3 g
Resazurin (0.1% fresh solution)	1 ml
Distilled water	To 1000 ml

v. Soya bean-casein digest medium

Formula: Table 4.6 describes formula of soya bean-casein digest medium.

Table 4.6: Formula of soya bean-casein digest medium

Ingredients	Quantity
Pancreatic digest of casein	17 g
Papaic digest of soya bean meal	3 g
Sodium chloride	5 g
Dibasic potassium phosphate	2.5 g
Dextrose	2.5 g
Distilled water	To 1000 ml

Procedure

- Dissolve the solids in distilled water by warming slightly to effect solution.
- Cool to the room temperature and add, if necessary, sufficient 0.1 M sodium hydroxide to give a final pH of 7.1 ± 0.2 after sterilization.
- Filter, if necessary, distribute into suitable containers and sterilize in an autoclave at 121°C for 20 minutes.
- Use soya bean-casein digest medium by inoculating it at 20–25°C under aerobic conditions.

It is valuable for detecting injured or other aerobic bacteria that grows slowly in the thioglycollate broth.

Precautions Against the Contaminations

The test for the sterility should be carried out in condition designed to avoid accidental contamination of the product during test using:

1. Test should be performed under a laminar sterile air flow unit.
2. Working condition in which the test is performed should be monitored regularly by sampling the air and surface of working area.
3. Adequate control test must be regularly performed.

Testing Procedures

1. Prescribed Quantity

Table 4.7 describes number of size of samples to be tested for sterility.

2. Incubation

a. Temperature

USP and European pharmacopoeia suggest 30–32°C for bacteria and 22°–25°C for lower fungi.

b. Time

The European pharmacopoeia recommended at least 7 days. USP for the steam sterilized product recommends 7 days and for other product preparation, it requires extension of 14 days. For aseptically processed product, tested by membrane filtration method, seven days incubation period is required.

The aim is to provide an adequate period for the recovery of organism suffering from the effect of heat or antibacterial agent and for the multiplication of these organisms.

c. Frequency of inspection

The container should be inspected every day because some bacteria produce a detectable turbidity at first but later settle as insignificant deposits at the bottom of the tubes and leave the clear uncontaminated broth above. Also, repeat test can be set up immediately after contaminant is detected.

Table 4.7: Size of samples to be tested for sterility

Quantity in each container preparation	Minimum quantity to be used for each culture medium
Liquids	
Less than 1 ml	Total contents of a container
1 ml or more but less than 40 ml	Half the contents of a container
40 ml or more but less than 100 ml	20 ml
100 ml or more	10% of the contents of a container but not less than 20 ml
Antibiotic liquids	1 ml
Other preparation soluble in water in isopropyl myristate	The whole content of each container to provide not less than 200 mg
Insoluble preparation, creams and ointments to be suspended or emulsified	The whole contents of each container to provide not less than 200 mg
Solids	
Less than 50 mg	Total contents of container
50 mg or more but less than 300 mg	Half the contents of a container
500 mg or more	100 mg
For catgut and other surgical sutures for veterinary use	3 sections of strands (each 30 cm long)
For surgical dressings/ cotton/gauze	100 mg per package
For sutures and other individually packed single use materials	The whole devices of material cut into pieces or disassembled

3. Interpretation of Results

If there is no sign of growth in any container, the sample and therefore the bulk or lot passes the test. If the growth is observed, all the previously mentioned tests are to be repeated with fresh samples. The repeat test is done to checkout that if the presence of contamination is because of faulty technique. So, repeat test should be carried out with exceptional care to prevent a recurrence of accidental contamination.

If no growth occurs in second test, it is believed that initial test was invalid and presence of contamination was due to inadequate test or faulty technique. If growth occurs in second test, European pharmacopoeia permit further repeat test using same testing procedure unless the same organism is found in the two sets. If no growth in third test, product passes the test. And if there is a growth, the organisms are isolated and identified.

If the contaminants are similar to first test, the product fails the test because if the same organism is recovered from two randomly selected batches of sample, it is assumed that product must be heavily contaminated. If contaminants are different, perform second retest using twice the number of sample by performing this retest, if there is no growth, product passes the test and if there is growth,, product fails the test.

Control Test

The result of the sterility test cannot relied upon if they can have any other explanation *except*:

1. In case of negative result, sterility of sample.
2. In case of positive result, contamination of sample. However, a negative result could also be due to:

   Inability of the broth to support the microbial growth because of

   i. Inadequate formulation

   ii. Accidental omission of any ingredient.

   iii. Overheating during the preparation and sterilization

   iv. In the aerobic media, failure to boil off oxygen from excessively oxygenated container.

3. Inhibition of the contaminants by a substance added in test. This could be a sample itself or a neutralizing agent used to destroy the antibacterial effect of ingredient of sample.

   Similarly, a positive result is due to:

   1. Lack of sterility of media.
   2. Accidental contamination during the testing.

Therefore the control test is necessary to show that these factors are not to be the explanation of the result.

1. Negative Control

In this no growth is expected. A container of medium from each batch used for the test is incubated at same time as the test container.

The control serves three purposes:

a. It conforms the medium is sterile.

b. It shows that the oxidation/reduction quality of indicators containing anaerobic medium is satisfactory.

c. It serves as a standard with which the corresponding test container can be compared during and after incubation.

Any substance other than sample added to test tube should be proved sterile by incubating suitable amount in appropriate media.

2. Positive Control (Fertility Test)

In these, growth is expected and sensitivity of media must be confirmed. Each type of medium is inoculated with an appropriate organism and after incubation under suitable condition, it is examined for growth. European pharmacopoeia suggests *Staphylococcus aureus* as aerobes, *Clostridium sphenoides* as anaerobes and *Candida albicans* as yeast. The medium must be shown capable of supporting growth of small number of bacteria in the presence of sample.

Inactivation of Antibacterial Substances

Many of pharmaceuticals that must be tested for sterility are contained medicament that can either destroy bacteria or prevent their growth. Other are preparation in which bactericides is included that is multi dose injection sterilized by heating with bactericide. When sample from these are added to test media, the concentration of antibacterial agent may be sufficient to prevent the bacterial growth and therefore prevent detection of contaminants.

It might be thought that these organisms could be ignored since, they are so successfully inhibited by the product but animal experiments shows that bacteria inhibited by certain antibacterial can become revived after injection because inhibitor is diluted by body fluid or neutralized by chemicals in tissue.

Three methods are used for this:

1. Inactivation by dilution

2. Inactivation by neutralization

3. Filtration

1. Inactivation by Dilution

The sample is added to a volume of medium sufficient to dilute the inhibitor to below its minimum bacteriostatic concentration.

The relationship between concentration of bactericide and rate at which it kills the microorganism is given by expression:

$$C^n . t = \text{Constant}$$

Where,

    C = Concentration of bactericide

    t = Time required to kill bacteria

    n = Dilution co-efficient indicates effect of dilution on rate of bactericidal infection.

Examples

a. Phenolic substances: Phenol, cresol, chlorocresol can be inactivated by adding 1 ml of sample to 50 ml of culture media. Dilution is done with medium only and not with extra agent.

b. Alcohol: Dilution is made by taking 1 ml of sample to 50 ml of test medium

c. Barbiturates: The substances are usually tested for sterility in dried state because injections are prepared immediately before use. 100 ml sample should be added to 100 ml of broth.

2. Inactivation by Neutralization

When dilution is impracticable, the sample is treated with a substance capable of neutralizing the inhibitor; the neutralizer must not be antibacterial itself. Inactivation by dilution is impracticable in two circumstances as follows:

i. When antibacterial agent has low dilution co-efficient. If this is 1 in above example, it requires only 20 min. to kill microbial population therefore very great dilutions are necessary to remove effect of this type of compound. They are impracticable because large volumes of broth are costly and they are difficult to manipulate. The test is less sensitive if sample size is smaller than relative volume of medium.

ii. When inhibitors are strongly adsorbed by or combine with bacterial cell wall.

Because of these two cases, inactivation by neutralization is more effective than dilution, e.g.

a. Mercurials

Mercurial compounds such as mercuric chloride, phenyl mercuric salt, thiomersal inhibit the bacteria by combining with sulfhydryl group of vital compound. Organisms may be apparently dead from exposure to mercuric chloride to be revived by treatment with ammonium sulphide. Mercury is removed from microorganism in the form of insoluble sulphide. All mercurials have less activity for bacterial metabolite than for certain other sulfhydryl compound and will leave former in preference for later with revival of inhibited cells. Most efficient revival is thioglycollate in concentration of 0.05%

b. Arsenicals

The antimicrobial arsenical compound that is neoarsphenamine, sulpharsphenamine, oxophenarsine are believed to act in same way as mercurials and inhibitory effect can be similarly neutralized by –SH compound. More amounts of Arsenicals are added in formulation (0.5%), and therefore, it requires more amount of sodium thioglycollate (0.4%).

c. Sulphonamides

They inhibit bacterial population by interfering with utilization of important growth factor PABA (p-aminobenzoic acid).

$$E + PABA \rightarrow E\ (PABA)$$

This is an essential step in the metabolism of the organism and antibacterial agent. In this case, sulphonamide, e.g. p-aminobenzene sulfonamide (PABS) can also combine with enzyme (E).

$$E + PABS \rightarrow E\ (PABS)$$

So that if adequate amount of E (PABA) will not be produced, metabolic chain will be broken, organism will be unable to grow and multiply. This type of antibacterial action is known as competitive inhibition, the fact is used in sterility testing for the preparation containing sulphonamides. PABA is added to broth to antagonize inhibitor and revive contaminants.

Low concentration is sufficient because enzyme having more affinity toward growth factor than for antagonist. Usually 5–10 mg/100 ml is added during preparation of N broth which is also known as PABA broth.

d. Quarternary ammonium compounds

Cetrimide, benzalkonium chloride, etc. are having detergent and antibacterial activity present in their complex cation. They are bacteriostatic in high dilutions. Because of their great surface activity, they are strongly absorbed on cell wall of microorganisms. Consequently it is not possible to use dilution method to overcome their effect and therefore, antagonist is necessary.

Anionic detergents such as soaps and sodium lauryl sulphate combine with this cation and precipitate the active cation of inhibitors. These anions are unsuitable because they have bacteriostatic activity themselves and very high concentration is required for full neutralization. One of the best antagonist is mixture of lecithin and a non-ionic surface active compound. Lecithin causes production of insoluble or feebly ionized complexes with quaternary or alteration in cell membrane making it less permeable. And non-ionic surfactants result in chemical bonding with inhibitors.

e. Chlorhexidine salts

They destroy bacterial cell by combining with cytoplasmic membrane and disrupting its structure and function. Lecithin is satisfactory inactivating agent. Broth containing 0.5% lecithin solubilized by non-ionic surface active agent is used.

f. Penicillin

Penicillinase inactivates penicillin by hydrolyzing β-lactum ring to produce penicilloic acid. It is used to prevent antibacterial action of benzyl, benzathine and procaine penicillins in culture media when preparation of these antibiotics is tested for sterility.

g. Other substances

Up to 0.2% methyl and 0.04% propyl ester of p-hydroxy-benzoic acid is inactivated by broth containing 5% polysorbate

80/20. 0.6% chlorbutol is inactivated by broth containing 5% polysorbate 20 and 10% polysorbate 80.

3. Separation from Inhibitors

When neither dilution nor neutralization is possible, contaminating organisms are separated from sample by filtration through bacterial proof filter. Contaminating organisms can be separated from the preparation to be tested, after washing, when becomes free from inhibitor, it is transferred on membrane on a suitable container of culture media.

Test for Sterility of Different Pharmaceutical Preparation as Per Indian Pharmacopoeia

There are two methods for test for sterility

Method I: Membrane filtration method

1. For aqueous solution
2. For liquids immiscible with aqueous vehicles and suspension
3. For oils and oily solutions
4. For ointments and creams
5. For soluble solids
6. For sterile devices

Method II: Direct inoculation method

1. For aqueous solution and suspension
2. For oils and oily solution
3. For ointments
4. For solids
5. For sterile devices

Method I: Membrane Filtration Method

This method needs exceptional skills and special knowledge.

Apparatus: A suitable unit consists of a closed reservoir and a receptacle between which a properly supported membrane of appropriate porosity is placed. A membrane generally suitable for sterility testing has a nominal pore size of not more than 0.45 ± 0.02 µm and diameter of approximately 47 mm and having edge of hydrophobic area about 3 mm wide. Preferably assemble and sterilize the entire unit with the membrane in place, prior to use.

Method of Test

1. For aqueous solution

Membrane is prepared by moistening with small quantity of suitable sterile solvent such as 0.1% w/v of neutral solution of meat or casein peptone (it renders the membrane less viable to damage and it decreases the retention of inhibitors). Take prescribed quantity of preparation and if necessary dilution is made with 100 ml of sterile diluents.

Transfer it to the membrane and filter immediately. For the solution having antimicrobial activity, wash the membrane by filtering 3–4 successive quantity of each of 100 ml of suitable sterile diluents (0.1% w/v of neutral solution of meat or casein peptone). After filtration, remove the membrane intact or divide into two parts. Immerse one part of membrane in 100 ml of soyabean casein digest medium and incubate at 20–25°C for not less than 7 days. Similarly, immerse the other half membrane in 100ml of fluid thioglycollate medium and incubate at 30–35°C for not less than 7 days.

2. For liquids immiscible with aqueous vehicles and suspension

Carry out the test prescribed under 'For aqueous solution'. For dissolving insoluble substance, sterile enzyme preparation such as penicillinase or cellulose may be added to 0.1% w/v of neutral solution of meat or casein peptone. If the substance under test contains lecithin, add polysorbate 80 to the above neutral solution and perform the test as described under 'For aqueous solution'.

3. For oils and oily solutions

Oils or oily solution of sufficient low viscosity may be filtered without dilution through a dry membrane (filter paper). Viscous oils may be diluted by sterile diluents such as isopropyl myristate that do not have antimicrobial property under condition of test. Allow the oil to penetrate the membrane and filter by applying pressure or suction gradually.

Wash the membrane by filtering through it with 3–4 successive quantity of each of approximately 100ml of suitable sterile diluents such as 0.1% w/v of neutral solution of meat or casein peptone that contain 0.1%w/v of polyethoxy ethanol or 0.1%w/v of polysorbate 80 (non-ionic surface active agent).

After filtration, remove the membrane intact or divide into two parts. Immerse one part of membrane in 100ml of soyabean casein digest medium and incubate at 20–25°C for not less than 7 days. Similarly, immerse the other half membrane in 100 ml of fluid thioglycollate medium and incubate at 30–35°C for not less than 7 days.

4. For ointments and creams

Dilute the ointments in a fatty base and emulsion of water in oil type with suitable sterile diluents such as isopropyl myristate (previously sterilized by filtration through a 0.22 μm membrane filter and that does not have antimicrobial property) to give a fluid concentration of 1% w/v. Heating is applied if necessary to not more than 40°C.

5. For soluble solids

Dissolve the prescribed quantity of substance being examined in a suitable sterile solvent such as 0.1% w/v of neutral solution of meat or casein peptone and carry out the test prescribed under 'For aqueous solution'.

6. For sterile devices

Aseptically transfer a sufficient volume of suitable sterile solvent such as 0.1% w/v of neutral solution of meat or casein peptone that contains 0.1% w/v of polysorbate 80 (non-ionic surface active agent) through the membrane so that the quantity recovered from each devices should not be less than 100 ml Filter the entire volume collected through membrane filter as described under 'for aqueous solution'.

Advantages of filtration technique

1. Wide application—they can be used for:
   a. Solution with or without inhibitory properties
   b. Soluble solids with or without inhibitory properties
   c. Insoluble solids without inhibitory properties
   d. Oils
   e. Ointments, for those, a non-inhibitory solvent or dispersing medium can be found
   f. Articles (e.g. syringes) that can be rinsed with a sterile fluid.

2. A large volume can be tested with one pad. Hence, the method is useful for testing the poorly soluble solids.

3. The volume of broth required is much smaller than that of testing by direct inoculation into culture media.

4. They are applicable for the substance for which no satisfactory inactivators are known, e.g. many antibiotics.

5. Some strongly adsorbed antibacterial agents (e.g. mercurials and quaternary ammonium compounds) can be treated with appropriate neutralizing solution and made inactivated on filter.

6. Sub culturing is often eliminated e.g. oils and oily preparation and substances like barbiturate give precipitates in broth.

Disadvantages of filtration technique

1. With membrane filters, the porosity of adsorption of sufficient medicament for test cannot be discounted entirely.

2. Highly skilled staff and exceptionally good aseptic technique are necessary.

Method II: Direct Inoculation Method

1. For Aqueous Solution and Suspension

Remove the liquid from the test containers by using sterile pipette or sterile syringe or a needle. Aseptically transfer the specified volume of material from each container to a vessel of culture medium. Mix the liquid with medium. Incubate the inoculated media unless otherwise specified in the monograph, at 30°–35°C in case of fluid thioglycollate medium and at 20°–25°C in case of soyabean casein digest medium for not less than 14 days. When the material to be examined produces the turbidity in a medium then the presence or absence of microbial growth cannot be determined readily by visual examination. In this case, transfer the suitable proportion of the medium to the fresh vessels containing the same medium between the third and seventh days after the test is started. Continue the incubation of transfer vessels for not less than 7 additional days after the transfer and for total of not less than 14 days.

2. For Oils and Oily Solution

Use the media containing 0.1% w/v of (4-tert-octylphenoxy) polyethoxy ethanol, 1% w/v of polysorbate 80 or other suitable emulsifying agent in an appropriate concentration that does not show any antimicrobial property. Carry out the test as described under 'for aqueous solution and suspension'.

3. For Ointments

Prepare the test media by diluting 10 folds in a sterile diluents such as 0.1% w/v solution of meat or casein peptone that contain 0.1% w/v solution of polyethoxy ethanol or 0.1% w/v of polysorbate 80 (non-ionic surface active agent) or any other aqueous vehicle capable of dispersing the test material homogeneously throughout the fluid mixture. Mix 10 ml of fluid mixture, so obtained with 80 ml of the medium and proceeds as directed under 'for aqueous solution and suspension'.

4. For Solids

Transfer the quantity of preparation to be examined to the prescribed quantity of medium and mix. The condition of incubation is same as that for the aqueous solution and suspension. When the material to be examined produces the turbidity in a medium then the presence or absence of microbial growth cannot be determined readily by visual examination. In this case, transfer the suitable proportion of the medium to the fresh vessels containing the same medium between the third and seventh days after the test is started. Continue the incubation of transfer vessels for not less than 7 additional days after the transfer and for total of not less than 14 days.

5. For Sterile Devices

For articles, that are having size and shape so as to permit complete immersion in not more than 1000 ml of culture medium—test the intact article using appropriate media and incubate as director under 'for aqueous solution and suspension'.

For transfusion and infusion assemblies, or where, the size of the article is such that the complete immersion of article is impracticable and only the fluid pathway must be sterile—flush the lumen of each of 20 units with a sufficient quantity of fluid thioglycollate medium and the lumen of each of 20 units with sufficient quantity of soyabean casein digest medium to give the recovery of not less than 15 ml of each medium and incubate with not less than 100 ml of each of 2 medias as directed under 'for aqueous solution and suspension'.

For devices in which the lumen is so small that the fluid thioglycollate medium will not pass through—substitute for fluid thioglycollate medium, i.e. alternative thioglycollate medium is used and incubate that inoculated medium anaerobically.

Other Sterility Test

Test for surgical dressings

Test for catgut and other surgical dressings

Test for paraffin gauze

Test for glassware

Test for equipment

Test for rubber and plastics sterility testing of air

1. Test for Surgical Dressings

The selected package is opened using aseptic precautions and appropriate portion is removed from three different portions of package. Table 4.8 describes number of size of samples to be tested for sterility.

The quantity of medium used should be sufficient to cover the selected portion of dressing. Sterility test can be achieved by filtration method. Shake each portion of dressing for 10 min with not less than 50 ml of suitable nutrient medium that contain 0.07% w/v of polysorbate 80 as a combining the microbial inactivating and washing solution.

Table 4.8: Number of size of samples to be tested for sterility	
Materials	*Minimum quantity to be used for each culture medium*
Absorbent cotton	Not less than 1 g
Woven material and adhesive dressing	About 10 cm^2
Cat gauze compress	1 complete compress

Then the washings are filtered as quickly as possible through membrane previously moistened with small amount of culture medium. Wash each membrane with not less than three successive 50 ml quantities of chosen sterile diluents. Membrane is transferred to the culture medium.

2. Test for Catgut and other Surgical Dressings

Open an appropriate number of packages using aseptic precaution and remove the suture. For each medium use five whole strands. When the sutures are presented in a multi strand package, the five strands required for each medium must be taken from the five different packages. Incubate for not less than 14–21 days.

Longer incubation time is required for following reasons:

1. Catgut is made from intestine of sheep whose slaughterhouse become heavily contaminated with spores of dangerous pathogens such as *Clostridium tetani* which is responsible for gas gangrene. During manufacturing, this may be trapped inside, which escapes the sterilization.
2. The incubation period of sterility is lengthened to 14–21 days because this gives time for culture media to penetrate the thread and organism should be recovered and multiplies in detectable turbidity.

3. Test for Paraffin Gauze

Modified fluid thioglycollate media containing 0.1% agar and 0.5% of gelatin, to increases the viscosity and to enhanced nutritive qualities, is used. The raised viscosity improves the dispersion of sample and reduces oxygenation during and after shaking. The medium is warmed up to about 52°C and the prescribed portions of dressings are inoculated into separate container. The leads are tightly reciprocating shaker for about 10 minutes. Afterwards the contents are allowed to cool in a slanting position and the resulting surface layer of congealed paraffin is broken by suitable shaker to ensure aerobic contamination during subsequent incubation.

After incubation at 32°C for 14 days, the jars are re-shaken for same time as before and 0.5 ml of sample is transferred to 50 ml volume of fresh medium, washed up to 50°C.

4. Test for Glassware

The glassware and apparatus like flasks, beakers, funnels, dropper bottles, glass rods, pipettes, petridishes, glass tubes, pestle and mortar, tiles, ointment tubes, ampoules, vials, syringes, needles, etc. may be sterilized either by moist heat or dry heat sterilization method but dry heat method is preferred. The glassware should be thoroughly cleaned with soap and hot water to remove grease and then rinsed with apyrogenic water.

New or very dirty articles should be soaked in cleaning solution overnight and then washed thoroughly. Then they are wrapped individually in a brown paper or suitable grade of paper so that the external surfaces should remain uncontaminated. The apparatus is not unwrapped until required for use. Flasks, beakers, tubes, pipettes, etc. should be plugged with long fiber non-absorbent cotton wool. The glassware so packed is kept on the shelves of the oven. Care must be taken that the articles are not tightly packed, there should be sufficient space in between the articles for the hot air to circulate. Contact with walls and floor of the oven must be prevented because these surfaces are hotter and may damage some of the articles and char the cotton wool plugs and paper wrappings. The usual recommended minimum holding temperature and time for glassware is 180°C for 11 minutes. When moist heat method is used it is essential that steam should come in contact with all the surfaces therefore a small quantity of water should be placed in the vessel otherwise they should be closed with a steam permeable closure. Sterilization is effected by heating at a temperature not lower than 160°C for 1 hour. There are chances that the glassware may discolor and darken in color if sterilized by ionizing radiation therefore it should not be applied.

5. Test for Equipment

Apparatus or devices that are made up of metal and surgical instruments, spatulas, metal part of bacterial filters such as Millipore filter; Seitz filter, etc. may be sterilized by steam under pressure at a temperature of 121°C for 15 to 30 minutes, depending upon the size of instruments. The material should be wrapped with muslin so that steam may penetrate to the surface of the metal parts. Sharp edged instruments should not be sterilized in hot air because long heating at the high temperature in hot air lead to oxidation which reduces the sharpness of the blades.

6. Test for Rubber and Plastics

Rubber articles such as stoppers, gloves, certain catheters and special feeding tubes may be sterilized in the autoclave at 121°C for 20 minutes. They must not be subjected to dry heat because high temperatures will spoil the rubber articles. Some synthetic rubbers such as silicon rubber has good heat resistance power therefore may be sterilized either by dry heat or moist heat. Rubber teats, stoppers and closures should be made of high-quality materials which should release negligible amounts of undesirable substances and absorb minimum amount of solutions in contact with them. For sterilization they should be first boiled with 5% solution of sodium carbonate for 30–60 minutes to remove sulphur and other impurities present in rubber during manufacturing process. Then they are thoroughly washed with hot water, wrapped sealed and sterilized in an autoclave at a temperature of 121°C for 20 minutes.

7. Sterility Testing of Air

The air is sterilized by the use of HEPA filters (High Efficiency Particulate Air filters). The air is supplied to clean room must be filtered through high-efficiency particulate air (HEPA) filters. The HEPA filter must be positioned at the inlet to the clean room and prefilter may be fitted upstream of the HEPA filter to prolong the life of the final filter. In these HEPA filters, use plated fiber glass paper as the filter medium. The filter consists of a continuous sheet of filtration material, plated with a corrugated separator placed between each plate and sealed into a rigid metal frame. Aluminium foil is used to form spacers in the HEPA filter.

Laminar air flow equipment

It can deliver clean air in a vertical, horizontal or curvilinear direction. The construction and directions of vertical and horizontal laminar airflow bench are shown in Fig. 4.7.

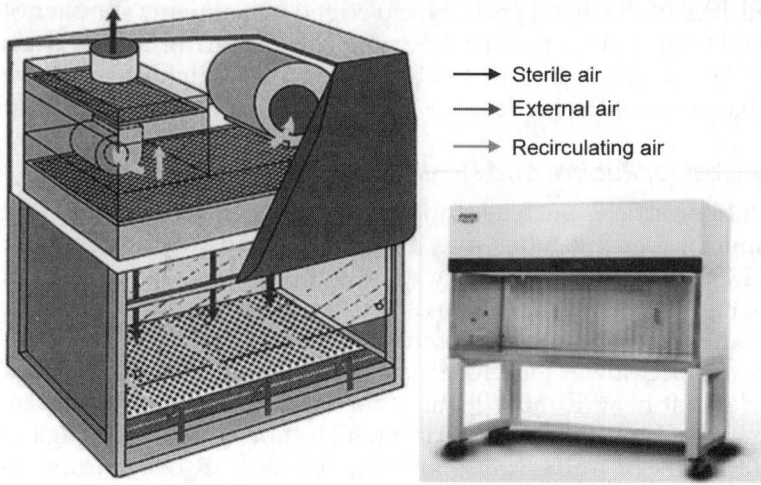

→ Sterile air
→ External air
→ Recirculating air

Fig. 4.7: Vertical laminar airflow cabinet

The air filtered from a laminar air flow is claimed to be 99.97% free from microbial contamination. This level is based upon the removal of dioctyl phthalate (DOP) particles of size 0.3 µm and large. Air velocity at all parts of the filter should be 90 ± 20 feet/min (0.54 m/sec)

Methods for sterility testing of air

It is necessary to monitor the area by suitable environmental control tests to provide the sterility conditions. These methods can be divided into general methods, air sampling methods and surface sampling methods which are given below.

a. General method

General methods are used to validate HEPA filter, detect particulate contamination and monitor the environment. These methods includes filter efficiency test, induction leak test, particulate contamination control test, air pressure test, air flow test, noise level tests, lighting test and temperature and humidity tests.

b. Air sampling methods

i. Electronic air particle counters: They are especially useful in determining the number of particle/microbes counts per cubic foot to classify the cleanliness of a particular room or area. Electronic counters count all particles/microbes but cannot differentiate between viable and non-viable microbes.

ii. Settle plates: A nutrient agar or other suitable medium is exposed to the atmosphere in the sampling area for predetermined period (20 to 60 minutes). Plates are incubated at 30°–35°C for 48 hours and colonies are counted. This is simple and inexpensive method commonly used for detection of microbial load in clean rooms. The major disadvantage of this method is the only those microorganisms that adheres to surface of the large particles are counted.

iii. Slit air sampler: It is one of the most widely used monitoring methods for manufacturing of parenterals and quality control environments. This is a device that collects viable airborne microbial and particulate contamination. Trypticase soy agar or any other suitable medium is placed on a circular plate in the slit air device and the cover containing the slit is secured above the agar plate. The speed of the plate rotation and the volume of air sampled can be adjusted to record the desired rate and degree of contamination of the all environment.

iv. Liquid impinge: The air sample may be drawn into a measured volume of nutrient broth in an impinger. Micro-organism in the broth, then may be collected by membrane filtration, incubated and counted.

v. Centrifugal air sampler (biotest): Airborne microorganisms approximately 16 inches above the sterile drum housing are drawn toward the impeller blades. By applying centrifugal forces, the microbial particles are impacted at high velocity onto the agar surface of the agar strip wound around the impeller blades. After incubation, colonies on the strips are counted and recorded.

c. Surface sampling method

i. Swab rinse test: This is a simple surface sample method in which sterile cotton swab tips to sample location. The swabs are then placed into tubes of culture media of sterile water (for microbial counting) and a sample of the water is placed on the solid agar plate.

ii. Rodac plates: Samples of the level of microorganisms on the surface can be determined by specially built convex surface petridish. With the rodac plates it is possible to roll low raised agar surface over flat or irregular surfaces to be tested. Surface contamination ban be quantified by counting the colonies after incubation at 30° to 35°C for 48 hours.

IV. MICROBIOLOGICAL ASSAY

Introduction

The microbiological or microbial assay is a type of biological assay in which the measurement of the relative potency or activity of a compound by determining the amount required for producing an anticipated effect on a suitable test under standard conditions. The biological assay refers to measurement of the relative potency or activity of compounds by determining the amount required to produce a specific, defined effect on a suitable test animal or organ under standard conditions. The biological assay may involve observations or measurement of effects obtained in any form of living matter, plant or animal. The term microbiological assay designates a type of biological assay, specifically, a biological assay performed with microorganisms, such as bacteria, yeasts and molds.

There are many agents who may either inhibit the growth of microorganisms, e.g. antibiotics, or may essential for their growth, e.g. vitamins and amino acids, can be standardized by microbiological assay. Microbiological assays measure the activity of antibiotics, or vitamins or amino acids that is to the extent of ability to inhibit or to support the growth of microorganisms, whereas chemical assays of such substance estimate only their potency, i.e. the concentration or amount. Hence, microbiological assays are of greater value in case of antibiotics, amino acids and vitamins.

Advantages of Microbiological Assay

1. It is used for those compounds which cannot be assayed by either physical or chemical assay method.
2. The methods are simple and rapid as compared to bioassay.
3. It reduces the mortality rate of animals.
4. Other than concentration, activity of the compounds can also be determined.

5. Accurate standardization of medicinal compounds can be achieved.

6. The naturally occurring therapeutic agents are assayed by this method

7. Use of large amount of sample and large number of instruments can be avoided.

Disadvantages of Microbiological Assay

1. Extreme sterile conditions should be maintained in the laboratory

2. It is time consuming method

3. Well trained, expert individuals are required to carry out microbial assay

4. Fluctuation in temperature or other condition during incubation may produce invalid result.

1. Microbiological Assay of Antibiotics

The inhibition of microbial growth under standardized conditions may be utilized for demonstrating the therapeutic efficacy of antibiotics. Any subtle change in the antibiotic molecule which may not be detected by chemical methods will be revealed by a change in the antimicrobial activity and hence microbiological assays are very useful for resolving doubts regarding possible change in potency of antibiotics and their preparations. The microbiological assay is based upon a comparison of the inhibition of growth of microorganism by measured concentrations of the antibiotics to be examined with that produced by known concentrations of a standard preparation of the antibiotic having a known activity.

Composition of the media used for microbiological assay of antibiotics

The ingredients required for the preparation of the test micro-organisms inoculums are shown in Table 4.9. Dissolve the ingredients in sufficient quantities of water to produce 1000 ml and add sufficient 1 M sodium hydroxide or 1 M hydrochloric acid, as required, so that after sterilization the pH is adjusted as given in Table 4.9. Various buffer solutions are given in Table 4.10.

Table 4.9: Composition of media: Quantities in g/1000 ml

Ingredients	A	B	C	D	E	F	G	H	I	J
Peptone	6	6	5	6	6	6	9.4	–	10	–
Pancreatic digest of casein	4	–	–	4	–	–	–	17	–	–
Yeast extract	3	3	1.5	3	3	3	4.7	–	–	–
Beef extract	1.5	1.5	1.5	1.5	1.5	1.5	2.4	–	10	15
Dextrose	1	–	1	1	–	–	10	2.5	–	–
Papaic digest of soya bean	–	–	–	–	–	–	–	3	–	5
Agar	15	15	–	15	15	15	23.5	12	17	15
Glycerin	–	–	–	–	–	–	–	–	10	–
Polysorbate 80	–	–	–	–	–	–	–	10	–	–
Sodium chloride	–	–	3.5	–	–	–	10	5	3	5
Dipotassium hydrogen phosphate	–	–	3.68	–	–	–	–	2.5	–	–
Potassium dihydrogen phosphate	–	–	1.32	–	–	–	–	–	–	–
Final pH (after sterilization)	6.5–6.6	6.5–6.6	6.95–7.05	7.8–8.0	7.8–8.0	5.8–6.0	6.0–6.2	7.1–7.3	6.9–7.1	7.2–7.4

Table 4.10: Buffer solutions

Buffer number	Dipotassium hydrogen phosphate (g)	Potassium dihydrogen phosphate (g)	pH adjusted after sterilization to
1	2	8	6 ± 0.1
2	16.73	0.523	8.0 ± 0.1
3	–	13.61	4.5 ± 0.1
4	20	80	6 ± 0.1
5	35	–	10.5 ± 0.1
6	13.6	4	7 ± 0.2

Standard and test solutions of antibiotics

The test solutions are prepared in concentration as shown in Table 4.11. Dissolve the quantity of the standard preparation of the given antibiotic in the solvent specified in Table 4.11.

Dilute the preparation to get required concentration as stated and stored in a refrigerator. At the same time prepare 3 control tubes, one containing the inoculated culture medium which is called as culture control and another identical with it but treated immediately with 0.5 ml of dilute formaldehyde solution, which is called as blank, and a third containing uninoculated culture medium. All the tubes will be placed in an incubator at the specified temperature as given in Table 4.11, for 4 to 5 hours. After incubation, add 0.5 ml of dilute formaldehyde solution to each tube. The growth of the test organism is measured by determining the absorbance of each of the solutions in the tubes against the blank.

Test organisms and preparation of inoculums

The test microorganisms for various antibiotics are shown in Table 4.12. The microorganism's suspensions are prepared by one of the following methods.

1. Maintain the test organism on slant of medium A and transfer to a fresh slant once a week. Incubate the slant at the specified temperature for 24 hours. Using 3 ml of saline solution wash the microorganism from the agar slant onto a large agar surface of medium A. Incubate for 24 hours at the appropriate temperature. Wash the growth from the nutrient surface using 50 ml of saline solution. Store the

Table 4.11: Preparation of standard and test solution of antibiotics

Antibiotics	Assay method	Solvent used	Final stock conc./ml	Median dose µg or units/ml of test solution
Amikacin	B	Water	1 mg	10 µg
Amphotericin B	A	Dimethyl formamide	1 mg	1 µg
Bleomycin	A	Buffer solution	2 units	0.04 units
Carbenicillin	A	Buffer solution	1 mg	20 µg
Doxycycline	B	0.1 M HCl	1 mg	0.1 µg
Erythromycin	A	Methano	1 mg	1 µg
Gentamicin	A	Buffer solution	1 mg	0.1 µg
Kanamycin sulphate	A	Buffer solution	800 unit	10 unit
	B	Water	1000 unit	1 unit
Neomycin	A	Buffer solution	1 mg	1 µg
Nystatin	A	Dimethyl formamide	1000 units	20 units
Rifampicin	A	Methanol	1 mg	5 µg
Streptomycin	A	Water	1 mg	1 µg
	B	Water	1 mg	30 µg
Tetracycline	A	0.1 M HCl	1 mg	2.5 µg
	B	0.1 M HCl	1 mg	0.24 µg

test microorganisms under refrigeration. Determine the dilution factor which will give 25% light transmission at about 530 nm. Determine the amount of suspensions to be added to each 100 ml of afar of nutrient broth by use of test plates or test broth. Store the suspension under refrigerator.

2. Proceed as given in method 1 but incubate the medium for 5 days. Centrifuge and decant the supernatant liquid. Resuspend the sediment with 50 to 70 ml of saline solution and heat the suspension for 30 minutes at 70°C. Wash the spore suspension 3 times with 50 to 70 ml of saline solution and heat the shock again for 30 minutes. Use test plates to determine the amount of the suspension required for 100 ml agar. Store the suspension under refrigeration. Maintain the test microorganism on 10 ml agar slant of

Table 4.12: Test microorganisms for various antibiotics

Antibiotic	Test organism	Method of assay
Amikacin	Staphylococcus aureus	B
Amphotericin B	Saccharomyces cerevisiae	A
Bacitracin	Micrococcus luteus	A
Bleomycin	Mycobacterium smegmatis	A
Carbenicillin	Pseudomonas aeruginosa	A
Doxycycline	Staphylococcus aureus	B
Erythromycin	Micrococcus luteus	A
Framycetin	Bacillus pumilus	A
	Bacillus subtilis	A
Gentamicin	Staphylococcus epidermidis	A
Kanamycin	Bacillus pumilus	A
sulphate	Staphylococcus aureus	B
Kanamycin B	Bacillus subtilis	A
Neomycin	Staphylococcus epidermidis	A
Novobiocin	Staphylococcus epidermidis	A
Nystatin	Saccharomyces cerevisiae	A
Oxytetracycline	Bacillus cereus var. mycoides	A
	Staphylococcus aureus	B
Polymyxin B	Bordetella bronchiseptica	A
Rifampicin	Bacillus subtilis	A
Streptomycin	Bacillus subtilis	A
	Klebsiella pneumoniae	B
Tetracycline	Bacillus cereus	A
	Staphylococcus aureus	B

medium G. Incubate at 32° to 35°C for 24 hours. Inoculate 100 ml of nutrient broth. Incubate for 18 to 24 hours at 37°C and proceed as described in method 1.

Two Official Pharmacopoeia Methods are Usually Employed

1. **Method A:** The cylinder-plate (or cup-plate) method
2. **Method B:** The turbidimetric (or tube assay) method

Method A: *The Cylinder-Plate (Or Cup-Plate) Method*

Principle

The cylinder-plate method depends upon diffusion of the antibiotic from a vertical cylinder through a solidified agar layer in a petridish or plate to an extent such that growth of the added microorganism is prevented entirely in a zone around the cylinder containing a solution of the antibiotic.

Procedure

Preparation of medium: Inoculate a previously liquefied medium appropriate to the assay (Tables 4.9 and 4.11) with the requisite quantity of suspension of microorganism. Add the suspension to the medium at a temperature between 40° and 50°C and immediately pour the inoculated medium into petridishes or large rectangular plates to give a depth of 3 to 4 mm (1 to 2 mm for nystatin).

Ensure that the layers of medium are uniform in thickness, by placing the dishes or plates on a level surface [21 ml base layer (uninoculated) + 4 ml seed layer (inoculated)]. The prepared dishes or plates must be stored in manner so as to ensure that no significant growth or death of test organism occurs before the dishes or plates are used and that the surface of the agar layer is dry at the time of use.

Preparation of sample and standard solution: Using the appropriate buffer solutions indicated in Tables 4.10 and 4.11, prepare solutions of known concentration of the standard preparation and solutions of corresponding assumed concentrations of the antibiotic to be examined. Where directions have been given in the individual monograph for preparing the solutions, these should be followed and further dilutions made with buffer solution as indicated in Table 4.11.

Apply the solutions of standard and sample to the surface of the solid medium in sterile cylinders or in cavities prepared in the agar. The volume of solution added to each cylinder or cavity, must be uniform and sufficient, almost to fill the holes when these are used. When petridishes are used, arrange the solutions of the standard preparation and the antibiotic to be examined on each dish so that they alternate around the dish and so that the highest concentrations of standard and test preparations are not adjacent. When plates are used, place the solutions in a Latin square design, if the plate is square, or if it is not, in a randomized block design. The same random design should not be used repeatedly.

Leave the dishes or plates standing for 1 to 4 hours at room temperature or at 4°C, as appropriate, as a period of pre-incubation diffusion to minimize the effects of variation in time between the applications of the different solutions. Incubate them for about 18 hours at temperature indicated in Table 4.11. Accurately measure the diameters or areas of the circular inhibition zones by using magnifying instrument zone reader and calculate the results by one of the following method.

1. One-level Assay with Standard Curve

Standard solution

Dissolve an accurately weighed quantity of the standard preparation of the antibiotic, previously dried where necessary, in the solvent specified in Table 4.11 and then dilute to the required concentration, as indicated, to give the stock solution.

Store in a refrigerator and use within the specified period indicated. On the day of assay, prepare from the stock solutions, five dilutions (S_1, S_2, S_3, S_4, and S_5) representing five test levels of the standard and increasing stepwise in the ratio of 4 : 5. Use the diluents specified in Table 4.11 and a sequence such that the middle or median has the concentration given in Table 4.11.

Sample solution

From the information available for the antibiotic preparation which is being examined (the unknown) assign to it an assumed potency per unit weight or volume and on this assumption prepare on the day of the assay a stock solution with the same solvent as used for the standard. Prepare from this stock solution a dilution to a concentration equal to the median level of the standard to give the sample solution.

Method

For preparing the standard curve, use a total of 12 petridishes or plates to accommodate 72 cylinders or cavities. A set of three plates (18 cylinders or cavities) is used for each dilution. On each of the three plates of the set fill alternate cylinders or cavities with solution S_3 (representing the median concentration of the standard solution) and each of the remaining 9 cylinders or cavities with one of the other four dilutions of the standard solutions. Repeat the process for the other three dilutions of the standard solution. For each unknown preparation use a set of three plates (18 cylinders or cavities) and fill alternate cylinders or cavities with the sample solution and each of the remaining nine cylinders of cavities with solution S_3. Incubate the plate for about 18 hours at the specified temperature and measure the diameters or the zones of inhibition.

Estimation of potency

Average the readings of solution S_3 and the readings of the concentration tested on each set of three plates, and average also all 36 readings of solution S_3. The average of 36 readings of solution S_3 is the correction point for the curve. Correct the average value obtained for each concentration (S_1, S_2, S_4 and S_5) to Fig. 4.8, it would be if the readings for the solution S_3 for that set of three plates were the same as correction.

Thus in correcting the value obtained with any concentration,

For example: Say S_1, If the average of 36 readings of S_3 is 18.0 mm average of the S_3 concentration on one set of three plates is 17.8 mm the correction is ± 0.2 mm If the average reading of S_1 is 16.0 mm the corrected reading of S_1 is 16.2 mm. Plot these corrected values including the average of the 36 readings for the solutions S_3 on 3-cycle semi log paper, using the concentrations in Units of µg/ml as the ordinate logarithmic scale (X-axis) and the diameter of the zones of inhibition as the abscissa (Y-axis).

Draw the straight response line either through these points by inspection or through the points plotted for the highest and lowest zone diameter obtained by means of the following expressions:

$$L = \frac{3a + 2b + c - e}{5}$$

$$H = \frac{3e + 2d + c - a}{5}$$

Where,

L = The calculated zone diameter for the lowest concentration of the standard curve response line

H = The calculated zone diameter for the highest concentration of the standard curve response line

c = Average zone diameter of 36 readings of the reference point standard solution

a, b, d, e = Corrected average values for the other standard solution, lowest to highest concentrations, respectively.

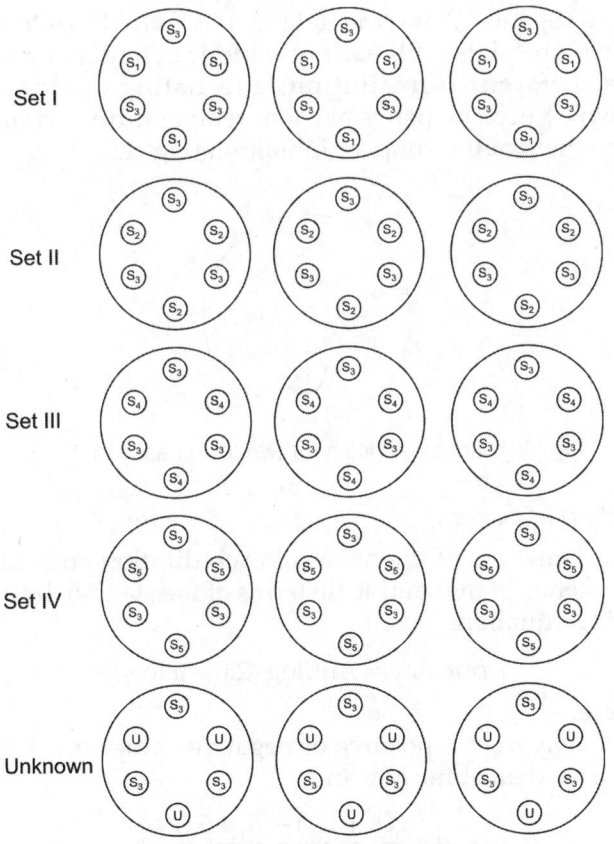

Fig. 4.8: Sets I to IV for the standard

Now, average the zone diameters for the sample solution and for solutions S_3 on the plates used for the sample solution. If the sample gives a large average zone size than the average of the standard solution S_3, add the difference between them to the zone size of the solution S_3 of the standard response line. If the sample zone size is smaller than the standard values, subtract the difference between them from the zone size of solution S_3 of the standard response line. From the response line, read the concentration corresponding to these corrected values of zone sizes.

2. Two-level Factorial Assay

Prepare parallel dilutions containing two levels of both the standard (S_1 and S_2) and the unknown (U_1 and U_2). On each of four or more plates, fill each of its four cylinders or cavities with a different test dilution, alternating standard and unknown. Keep the plates at room temperature and measure the diameters of the zones of inhibition (Fig. 4.9).

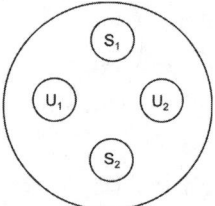

Fig. 4.9: Set of petridish for two-level assay method

Estimation of potency

Sum of diameters of the zones of each dilution and calculate the % potency of the sample (in terms of the standard) from the following equation:

$$\% \text{ potency} = \text{Antilog} (2.0 + a \log I)$$

Where,

> a = may have a positive or negative value and should be used algebraically and

$$a = \frac{(U_1 + U_2) - (S_1 + S_2)}{(U_1 + U_2) + (S_1 - S_2)}$$

Where,

U_1 and U_2 = The sums of the zone diameters with solutions of the unknown of high and low levels

S_1 and S_2 = The sums of the zone diameters with solutions of the standard of high and low levels

I = Ratio of dilutions

If the potency of the sample is lower than 60% or greater than 150% of the standard, the assay is invalid and should be repeated using higher or lower dilutions of the same solution.

The potency of the sample may be calculated from the expression

$$\frac{\% \text{ potency} \times \text{assumed potency of the sample}}{100}$$

3. Other Designs

1. Factorial assay containing parallel dilution of three test levels of standard and the unknown.
2. Factorial assay using two test levels of standard and two test levels of two different unknowns.

Method B: Turbidimetric Or Tub Assay Method

Principle

It depends upon the inhibition of growth of microbial culture in a uniform solution of the antibiotic in a fluid medium that is favorable to its rapid growth in the absence of the antibiotics.

Advantage

Shorter incubation period for the growth of the test organism (usually 3 to 4 hours).

Disadvantages

1. The presence of solvent residue or other inhibitory substance affects this assay more than cylinder plate-assay.
2. Care should be taken to ensure freedom from such substances in the final test solutions.
3. This method is not recommended for cloudy or turbid preparations. As the concentration increases, turbidity decreases because growth decreases.

Procedure

Prepare 5 different concentration of the standard solution for preparing the standard curve by diluting the stock solution of the standard preparation of the antibiotic (Table 4.11) and increasing stepwise in the ratio 4 : 5. Select the median concentration (Table 4.11) and dilute the solution of the substance being examined (unknown) to obtain approximately this concentration. Place 1 ml of each concentration of the standard solution and of the sample solution (Figs 4.10 to 4.12).

At the same time prepare three control tubes, one containing the inoculated culture medium (culture control), and another identical with it but treated immediately with 0.5 ml of dilute formaldehyde solution (blank) and a third containing uninoculated culture medium. Place all the tubes, randomly

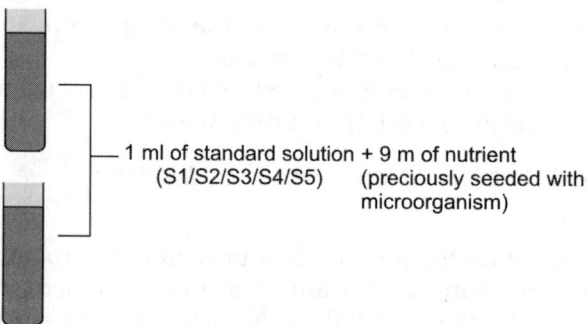

1 ml of standard solution + 9 m of nutrient
(S1/S2/S3/S4/S5)   (preciously seeded with
                     microorganism)

Fig. 4.10: Standard sample tube

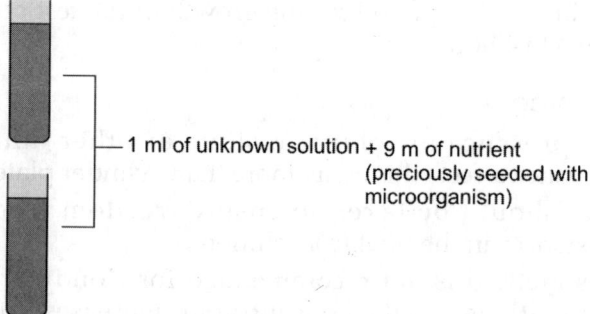

1 ml of unknown solution + 9 m of nutrient
                     (preciously seeded with
                     microorganism)

Fig. 4.11: Unknown sample tube

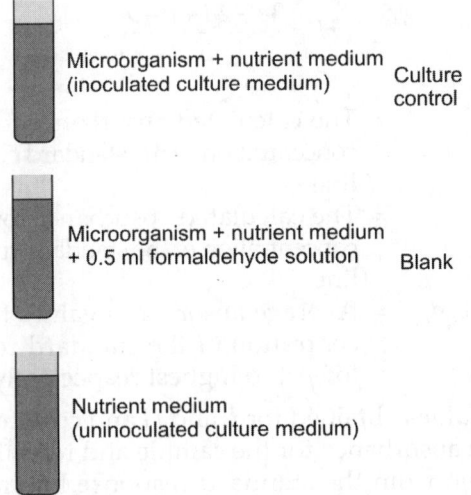

Microorganism + nutrient medium
(inoculated culture medium)   Culture control

Microorganism + nutrient medium
+ 0.5 ml formaldehyde solution   Blank

Nutrient medium
(uninoculated culture medium)

Fig. 4.12: Tubes containing culture control, blank and uninoculated culture medium

distributed or in a randomized block arrangement, in an incubator or a water-bath and maintain them at the specified temperature (Table 4.11) for 3 to 4 hrs.

After incubation add 0.5 ml of dilute formaldehyde solution to each tube. Set the spectrophotometer at zero absorbance with clear, uninoculated broth prepared as specified or the particular antibiotic including the same amount of test solution and formaldehyde as found in each sample. Measure the growth of the test organism by determining the absorbance at about 530 nm of each of the solutions in the tubes against the blank.

Estimation of potency

Plot the average absorbance for each concentration of the standard on semi-logarithmic paper with the absorbents on the arithmetic scale (Y-axis) and concentration on the logarithmic scale (X-axis). Construct the best straight response line through the points either by inspection or by means of the following expressions:

$$L = \frac{3a + 2b + c - e}{5}$$

$$H = \frac{3e + 2d + c - a}{5}$$

Where,

L	= The calculated absorbance for the lowest concentration of the standard curve response line
H	= The calculated absorbance for the highest concentration of the standard curve response line
a, b, c, d, e	= Average absorbance values for each concentration of the standard response line lowest to highest respectively.

Plot the values obtained for L and H and connect the points. Average the absorbance for the sample and read the antibiotic concentration from the standard response line multiply the concentration by the appropriate dilution factors to obtain the antibiotic content of the sample.

2. Precision of Microbiological Assay

i. The fiducial limit or error of the estimated potency should be not more than 105% and not less than 95% of the estimated potency unless otherwise stated in the individual monograph.

ii. Dynamics of zone formation.

iii. During the incubation, the antibiotic diffuses from the reservoir and that part of microbial population which is away from the influence of antibiotic increases by cell division.

iv. The edge of the zone is formed when the minimum concentration of antibiotic which will inhibit the growth of organisms on the plate.

v. The position of zone edge is determined by initial population density, growth rate of organism and rate of diffusion of antibiotic.

vi. Pre-incubation increases the number of microorganism on the plate and so critical population density is achieved rapidly and so zones will be smaller.

vii. Decrease the microbial growth rate gives the larger zones of inhibition.

viii. Increase in the sample size or decrease in agar thickness, increase the zone size.

ix. Thus when designing an assay, indicator organism, medium, sample size, incubation temperature, etc. should be optimized to give a large range of zone sizes over the required range of antibiotic concentration.

x. Zone size depends upon sample size, agar thickness, organism population density, organism growth rate, and drug diffusion rate.

3. Microbiological Assay of Vitamins

Certain microorganisms require vitamin or amino acids (factor) for their normal growth and are sensitive to very small amounts of the required factor. It is ability of these organisms (test organism) to synthesize the factor being assayed that forms the basis of the microbiological assay of vitamins and amino acids. Thus the test organism is inoculated in the special media which are nutritionally complete in all respects except for the actor under study. This serves as the control in which no or minimal growth of microorganisms is exhibited. In another set, graded amounts of factor (dose) are added and the growth of test organism (response) is observed. Usually the response (growth of the test organism) is proportional to the dose (amount of factor) added to the medium.

i. Microbiological assay of calcium pantothenate

The reagents required and the method used for the micro-biological assay of calcium pantothenate are applied below:

Test microorganisms

For this assay, the *Lactobacillus plantarum* is used as a test microorganism.

Medium

Table 4.13 describes formulations of media for assay of calcium pantothenate.

It is prepared by dissolving the anhydrous dextrose and sodium acetate in previously mixed solutions and the pH is adjusted with 1 N NaOH to a value of 6.8. Finally, it is diluted to 250 ml with water and mixed.

Table 4.13: Formulations of media for assay of calcium pantothenate

Acid hydrolyzed casein solution	25 ml
Cystine tryptophan solution	25 ml
Polysorbate 80 solution	0.25 ml
Dextrose anhydrous	10 g
Sodium acetate, anhydrous	5 g
Adenine-guanine-uracil solution	5 ml
Riboflavin-thiamine-HCl-biotin solution	5 ml
p-amino benzoic acid-niacin-pyridoxine hydrochloride solution	5 ml
Salt solution A	5 ml
Salt solution B	5 ml

Standard stock solution of calcium pantothenate

Each ml of this solution contains 50 µg of calcium pantothenate. It is prepared by dissolving 50 mg of calcium pantothenate in about 500 ml of water; 10 ml of 0.2 N acetic acid and 100 ml of 1.6 %w/v of solution of sodium acetate are added and volume is made up to 1000 ml by adding sufficient water. This solution is stored under toluene in a refrigerator.

Standard solution

Standard solution contains 0.04 µg of a pantothenate per ml prepared by diluting standard stock solution with water.

Test solution

Test solution prepared in water should contain approximately 80 ml concentration.

Method

Standard solution (1, 2, 3, 4 and 5 ml) is added to test tubes in duplicate. To each test tube and to another 4 similar tubes containing no standard solution, 5 ml of medium solution are added and volume is made up to 10 ml with water. In another step, volumes of test solution corresponding to 3 or more level as taken above are added to similar test tubes in duplicate. To each tube, add 5 ml of medium solution and volume is made up to 10 ml with water.

One complete set of standard and assay tubes together is placed in one rack and the duplicate set is kept in a second rack. Tubes of both series are heated in an autoclave at 121°C for 5 minutes, cooled; 1 drop of inoculums is added to each tube except two of the four tubes containing no standard solution, i.e. blank and mixed. The tubes are incubated at a temperature between 30° and 37°C for 16 to 24 hrs. Transmittance of the tubes is measured in the spectrophotometer at a specific wavelength between 540 and 660 nm.

Calculation

A standard concentration-response curve is prepared by plotting the transmittance against the log of the ml of standard solution per tube. The response is calculated by adding together the two transmittances for each level. Calcium pantothenate concentration in the test sample is determined with the help of standard concentration-response curve.

ii. Microbiological assay of Niacin (Niacinamide)

Test organism

The organism to be selected must be able to utilize free niacin, niacinamide, nicotinic acid, cozymase and niacinamide nucleoside. *Lactobacillus plantarum* fully satisfy this requirement. This organism is also non-pathogenic, easy to culture and least offered by the presence of other stimulatory or inhibitory substances normally found in the pharmaceutical preparations containing niacin. It may be grown on a simple stab culture. The range of 0.05 to 0.5 µg of niacin per tube can be used.

Standard niacin stock solution

It contains 100 µg/ml of USP niacin reference standard which is further diluted to concentration of 10 µg/ml both water.

Standard niacin solution

It contains between 10 ng to 40 ng of niacin per ml and is prepared from standard stock solution by dilution with water.

Test solutions

The sample can be extracted either in acid or alkali medium by addition of alkali or acid such that the final volume contains 0.1 g of niacin per ml.

Basal medium

Table 4.14 describes formulations of media for assay of niacin (niacinamide).

Table 4.14: Formulations of media for assay of niacin (niacinamide)	
Acid hydrolysed casein solution	25 ml
Cystine tryptophan solution	25 ml
Dextrose anhydrous	10 g
Sodium acetate, anhydrous	5 g
Adenine-guanine-uracil solution	5 ml
Riboflavin-thiamine-HCl-biotin solution	5 ml
p-amino benzoic acid-niacin-pyridoxine hydrochloride solution	5 ml
Salt solution A	5 ml
Salt solution B	5 ml

Method

Standard solution (1, 2, 3, 4 and 5 ml) is added to test tubes in duplicate. To each test tube and to another four similar tubes containing no standard solution, 5 ml of medium solution are added and volume is made up to 10 ml with water. In another step, volumes of test solution corresponding to three or more level as taken above are added to similar test tubes in duplicate.

To each tube, add 5 ml of medium solution and volume is made up to 10 ml with water. One complete set of standard and assay tubes together is placed in one rack and the duplicate set is kept in a second rack. Tubes of both series are heated in an autoclave at 121°C for 5 minutes, cooled; 1 drop of inoculums is added to each tube except two of the four tubes containing no standard solution, i.e. blank and mixed.

The tubes are incubated at a temperature between 30° and 37°C for 16 to 24 hrs. Transmittance of the tubes is measured in the spectrophotometer at a specific wavelength between 540 and 660 nm.

Calculation

Standard curve is prepared. From this curve, concentration of the test sample is determined by interpolation. If the results are to be expressed as niacinamide instead of niacin, then the values obtained are multiplied by 0.992

iii. Microbiological assay of vitamin B_{12} (cyanocobalamin)

The basic medium used for the assay of vitamin B_{12} activity is quite complex and contains a variety of essential components as a mixture in solution. One set of tubes contains measured amounts of a standard cyanocobalamin solution and graded volumes of the test sample (unknown) are added to another corresponding set of tubes. All the tubes are inoculated with a small amount of culture of *Lactobacillus leichmannii* and then inoculated. The extent of growth is determined by measure the light transmittance in a spectrophotometer. Transmittance values (response) for different concentration (dose) of standard cyanocobalamin solution are used to obtain the concentration response curve. The amount of vitamin B_{12} present in the test sample is calculated from the standard curve by interpolation.

4. Microbiological Assay of Amino Acids

Accurate methods for the quantitative determination of amino acids are not available. Procedures involving elution from paper chromatograms have shown poor reproducibility and low recovery rates and the column chromatography method of Moor and Stein requires expensive equipment.

Test organisms

Streptococcus faecalis is used for the assay of both valine and leucine and *Leuconostoc mesenteroides* for methionine.

Media

The test organisms are maintained as stab cultures in *Bacto-lactobacilli* agar at 4°C. A 24 hour old culture in 10 ml *Bacto-lactobacilli* broth is centrifuged and the deposit obtained by centrifugation is re-suspended in 20 ml of sterile saline. 0.5 ml of suspension is made up to 20 ml with sterile saline. The inoculums consist of one drop of this final suspension. The appropriate Bacto-amino acid assay medium is used for the actual assay.

Amino acid solutions

Earlier, L-form of valine and DL-form of methionine and leucine were used. But more recently the L-forms of all three amino acids have been used. 100 mg of L-valine and L-leucine and 50 mg of L-methionine are dissolved in separate 100 ml quantities of distilled water of AR purity. The working solutions are prepared by diluting 1 ml of the above solutions to 100 ml (valine and leucine) or 200 ml (methionine) with distilled water. This gives a final concentration of 10 µg/ml (valine and leucine) and 2.5 µg/ml (methionine).

Apparatus

The assay tubes consist of Pyrex test tubes measuring 150 × 16 mm fitted with aluminum caps. New unused sterile universal containers are used for the collection of blood and for the storage of culture media and sera. All glassware is chemically cleaned before sterilization. Control sera were obtained in about 200 ml quantities from the Welsh Regional Blood Transfusion Center. Normal sera were obtained from healthy volunteers, mainly hospital staff, and from a small number of healthy patients undergoing minor surgery. To ensure as constant metabolic state as possible, all vein punctures were done immediately before the subjects received their mid-day meal. All sera were stored at –20°C.

De-proteinization

There are 2 methods for obtaining a protein-free filtrate, i.e. precipitation by acetic acid and ultrafiltration. In the former method, 3 ml of 0.05 N acetic acid is added to 3 ml of serum. 9 ml of distilled water is added and the mixture placed in a boiling water bath for 3 to 5 minutes and filtered. The pH of the filtrate is adjusted to that of the assay medium (6.8). 1 ml and 2 ml quantities of the filtrate equivalent to 0.2 ml and 0.4 ml of serum are used in each assay. Serum is ultrafiltered overnight through 8/32 inch cellophane dialysis tubing, one end of which is sealed and the other end is connected to a compressed air cylinder from which a pressure of 10 lb/square inch is maintained.

Assay procedure

Increasing amounts of standard solution of the amino acid to be assayed are placed in the assay tubes. Each serum is assayed at two different dilutions. All tubes are set-up in triplicate and

2 ml of double strength appropriate amino acid assay medium is added to each. After autoclaving at 10 lb pressure for 10 minutes, each tube is inoculated with the appropriate test organism and all are then incubated at 37°C for 17 hours.

After thorough shaking the optical densities of the resulting growths and inoculated blank (tube 1 in which there is no growth, due to the lack of an essential amino acid) are measured against water in an Optica CF4 spectrophotometer using 1 cm cuvettes ate 600 mµ. The optical density of each triplicate set of tubes after subtracting the blank is plotted against the amino acid content per tube.

Results

Acid precipitation of protein compared with serum ultrafiltration: As acid precipitation of protein involved heating the protein in an acid solution, it was thought advisable in view of the high degree of sensitivity of the method of amino acid assay employed to establish whether minute quantities of amino acids might be liberated as the result of minimal protein hydrolysis. Valine was therefore assayed in 3 sera on 3 different occasions, each after deproteinization by acid precipitation and also after ultrafiltration. The results obtained as there is no significant difference in the serum amino acid level following the two methods of deproteinization the acid precipitation method was used in the rest of the work.

IMPORTANT STUDY QUESTIONS

1. Enlist methods for sterility testing. Discuss direct inoculation method. (Dec 2010)

2. **Explain:** Sterility, SAL, Incineration, MIC, zone of inhibition. (Dec 2010)

3. Describe cup-plate method for microbiological assay. (Dec 2010, June 2011)

4. Explain microbiological assay. Name microbes used in assay of: Amphotericin B, Erythromycin, Carbenicillin, Rifampicin, Tetracycline. (Dec 2010)

5. Discuss microbiological assay of Cyanocobalamin. (Dec 2010)

6. **Explain:** Total count and Viable count. Describe photometric method for determining total count. (Dec 2010)

7. Why test for sterility is carried out? What is the importance of control test in the test for sterility? (June 2011)

8. Discuss the principle underlying microbiological assay of vitamins. (June 2011)

9. Classify the various methods of bacterial counts. Discuss the plate count technique. (June 2011)

10. How do perform test for sterility of sodium sulphacetamide eye drops. (June 2011)

11. Why is bacterial count carried out in Pharma industry? (Dec 2011)

12. Describe any one method for assay of antibiotics. (Dec 2011)

13. How is the test for sterility of catgut carried out? (Dec 2011)

14. Discuss the test for surgical dressings and sterile devices.

15. Enlist the methods for microbiological assay. Describe in brief about turbidimetric/tube assay method.

16. Discuss the microbiological assay of vitamins.

17. Discuss the microbiological assay of amino acids.

Bibliography

1. A textbook of Microbiology, P. Chakraborty, New Central Publication, 2001.

2. A textbook of Microbiology, R. C. Dubey, S. Chand Publication, 2005.

3. General Microbiology, Roger Y. Stainer, fifth edition, Macmillan Press Ltd, Hampshire, 1986.

4. Indian Pharmacopoeia 2010, Government of India, Ministry of Health and Family welfare, The Indian Pharmacopoeia Commission, Ghaziabad.

5. Microbiology concepts and application, Paul A. Ketchum, John Wiley and Sons. Inc., 1988.

6. Microbiology, Lansing M. Prescott, Fifth edition, The McGraw-Hill Companies, 2002.

7. Microbiology, Michael J. Pelczar, Fifth edition, Tata McGraw-Hill Publication Limited.

8. Modern Industrial Microbiology and Biotechnology, Nduka Okafor, Science publisher, New Hampshire, 2007.

9. Pharmaceutical Microbiology, Ashutosh Kar, New Age International Publishers, 2008.

10. Pharmaceutical Microbiology, Hugo and Russel, Seventh edition, Black Well publishing limited, Oxford U.K, 2004.

11. Textbook of Microbiology, R Ananthanarayan, sixth edition, Orient Longman Limited, 2000.

12. World of Microbiology and Immunology, Bringham Narins, Volume 1 & 2, Thomson Gale Inc., 2003.

Index

Acidophiles 57, 92
Acridine dyes 155, 156
Actinomycetes 20, 46, 53, 57–59,
        79, 83, 128
Aerobic bacteria 55, 91, 93,
        94, 108, 233
Agar plate method 190, 191
Alcohols 13, 150, 151, 185
Aldehydes 158
Algae 11
Alternatively
        thioglycollate media 231
Anaerobic
    bacteria 55, 91, 94, 108, 226
    chamber 95
    jar 96, 97
Analytical microbiology 210, 211
Animal virus 20, 112, 117
Antimicrobial agent 131
Antiseptic 131
Archaea 2, 10
Arsenicals 239
Aseptic techniques 185
Atomic force microscopy (AFM) 41
Autoclave 165
Autotrophs 55, 92
Avirulent 115, 121

Bacilli 52
Bacteria 2, 10
Bacterial virus 20, 112, 121
Bacteriophage 114

Bacteriostasis 131
Berkefeld filters 179
Binary fission 102
Biological indicator 207
Bowie-Dick test 206
Breed's method 211, 212
Bright field microscope 23
Browne's tubes 205
Budding 103

Capsid and envelope 113
Capsule 48, 75
Cathode rays 174
Cell
    activity 211, 212, 222
    count 211, 212
    culture 119
    inclusions 81
    mass 211
Centrifugal air sampler/
        biotest 251
Chemical
    disinfectant 147
    dosimeter 206
    indicator 205, 206
Chemotrophs 55
Chick-Martin test 195, 197
Chlorhexidine salts 240
Chlorine and chlorine
        compounds 152
Classification of
    stains 42
    virus 110

Cocci 52, 53
Complex viruses 112
Conductivity method 216
Confocal microscopy 34
Conidiospores 104
Continuous
    cell lines 120, 122
    growth 102
Control test 236
Copper 155
Coulter counters method 211
Counting chamber method 213
Cultivation of plant viruses 20, 121
    aerobic bacteria 93
    anaerobic bacteria 94
    autotrophs 92
    bacteriophage/
        bacterial virus 121
    heterotrophs 93
    viruses 117
Cup plate method 191, 258
Cylinder plate method 258

D value 134
Dark field microscope 23, 26
Death rate of microorganisms 134
Decimal reduction time 134
Decline or death phase 99
De-proteinization of
        amino acids 272
Desiccation 170
Determination of cell
    activity 222
    count 212
    mass 220
    nitrogen content 220
Diauxic growth 101
Differential
    interference contrast
        microscopy 23, 30
    staining technique 45

Diploid cell strains 119
Direct
    inoculation method 241, 244
    microscopic count 212
Disinfectant 131
Ditch-plate technique 194
Dry
    heat sterilization 162, 204
    weight measurement 212, 220
Dyes 155
Dynamics of disinfection 138

Edward Jenner 6
Electron
    beam radiation 162, 174
    microscopy 35
Electronic
    air particle counters 250
    enumeration of cell
        number 211, 214
Embryonated egg 117
Endo flagella 68
Endospore (spore) staining 48
Endospore 48, 83
Enveloped virus 112
Errors in counting 223
Evaluation of disinfectants 189
Explants culture 119
Exponential phase 98, 99
Extinction time methods 195

Factors
    affecting the disinfectant
        action 138
    affecting the thermal
        destruction 136
Facultative
    anaerobic bacteria 56
    thermophiles 57
Fertility test 237
Fimbriae 73

Flagella 68
  staining 49
Fluid thioglycollate medium 229
Fluorescence microscopy 32
Fragmentation 102, 103
Fungi 2, 11

Gamma rays 162, 174
Gaseous agents 159
Germicide 131
Germs 2
Glycocalyx 74
Gradient plate method 193
Gram-negative cell wall 60
Gram-positive cell wall 75
Gram staining 45
Growth cycle of bacteria 98

Halogens 151
Heat sensitive tape 206
Heating with a bactericide 168
Heavy metals and
          their compounds 154
Helical viruses 110
Heterotrophs 55
Hot
   air oven 161, 163
   air sterilization 163

Icosahedral virus 110
Incineration 162
Indirect (relief) staining 43
Intuitive method 49
In-use test 201
Isolation
   and identification of
            viruses 127
   of bacteria 104
   of microbes 104

John Tyndall 6

Kelsey-Sykes method 195, 201

Lag phase 98, 99
Laminar air flow equipment 249
Latin hairs 73
Life cycle of bacteriophages 20, 121
Light microscopy 23
Lithotrophs 55
Log phase 99
Lysogenic 115
Lytic cycle 115, 121

Mechanical sieving 182
Membrane
   filter count 212, 219
   filters 177, 181
   filtration method 241
Mercurials 239
Mesophiles 57, 91
Mesosomes 81
Methods of microbial count 211
Microbial counts 211
Microbiological
   antibiotics 253
   assay of amino acids 271
   assay 252
   calcium pentothanate 267
   niacin (niacinamide) 269
   vitamin B_{12}/cyanocoba-
      lamin 271
   vitamins 267
Millipore filter 181
Moist heat sterilization 165
Monochrome staining 44
Motility 72
Multicellular animal parasites 12
Mycoplasmas 53

Negative
   control 236
   staining 43
   staining for capsules 47
Nephelometric method 221

Neutrophils 57
Non-stringent/tolerant
    anaerobes 56
Nucleoid 82
Numerical taxonomy 49
Nutrient media required for
    growth 87
Nutritional requirement
    of virus 116

One level assay 259
Organ culture 119
Organotrophs 55
Osmotic pressure 92, 171

Packed cell volume 211, 216
Pasteurization 169
Penicillin 240
Peptidoglycan 76
Phase contrast microscope 28
Phenol and phenolic
    compound 147
Phenol coefficient test 200
Photometric method 212, 221
Physical indicator 204
Pili 73
Plant virus 112
Plasma membrane 75
Plasmid 82
Plate-count method 217
Polyhedral virus 110
Positive control 237
Pour plate method 105
Precautions against the
    contamination 234
Precautions for
    handling of sterilization
    equipment 188
Precision of microbiological
    assay 266
Prereduced media 94

Primary cell cultures 119
Prokaryotic and
    eukaryotic protists 3
Proportional count method 215
Prototroph 55
Protozoa 66

Quarternary ammonium
    compounds 157, 240

Radiation sterilization 161, 172
Reproduction of bacteria 102
Ribosomes 81
Rickettsia 63
Rideal Walker test 195, 196
Robert Koch 9
Rodac plates 252
Roll tube method 104, 107
Royce sachet 206

Sample size 226
Sampling 225
Sanitizer 132
Sarcinae 54
Scanned probe microscopy 40
Scanning
    electron microscope 35, 38
    tunneling microscopy 41
Seitz filter 177
Selection of the samples 226
Semi-fluid hydrosulphite
    medium 232
Sensitivity 226
Separation from inhibitors 241
Serial dilution in
    fluid media 190
    solid media 190
Silver 155
Simple staining 43
Sintered glass filter 177, 178
Sources of contamination 185

Soya bean-casein digest
          medium 233
Special staining 47
Spirochetes 53, 65
Spontaneous generation of
          organisms 5
Sporangiospores 102
Spread plate method 106
Staining technique 41
Standard and test solutions
          of antibiotics 255
Standardization and
          testing of filters 183
Stationary phase 99, 100
Steam under pressure 161, 165
Sterility testing of air 249
Sterilization 161
     by filtration 175
     of vaccines 170
Streak plate method 104
Stringent/strict anaerobes 56
Structure of virus 113
Sulphonamides 239
Surface
     film test 195, 200
     sampling method 251
Suspension test 195, 196
Swab rinse test 251
Synchronous growth 20, 100
Synthetic detergents 157

Teichoic acid 76
Temperate 115
     cycle 121, 125
Theories of staining 42

Thermal
     death time 134
     resistance of microorganisms 133
Thermophiles 57
Thioglycollate broth
          medium 231, 232
Tissue culture 117, 119
Total count 211, 212
Transmission electron
          microscope 35, 36
Trichomes 54
Triphenylmethane 155, 156
True/obligate/steno
          thermophiles 57
Tube
     assay method 257
     dilution test 190
Turbidimetric method 212, 221
Two-level factorial assay 262
Tyndallization 161, 168

United States Food and
          Drugs method 195, 198

Validation 203
Viable count 212, 216
Vibrios 52
Virulent 115
Viruses 109

Whittaker's five kingdom
          concept 4
Witness tubes 206
Wright's method 211, 215

X-rays 162, 174